How to Cure the *Plague*
& Other Curious Remedies

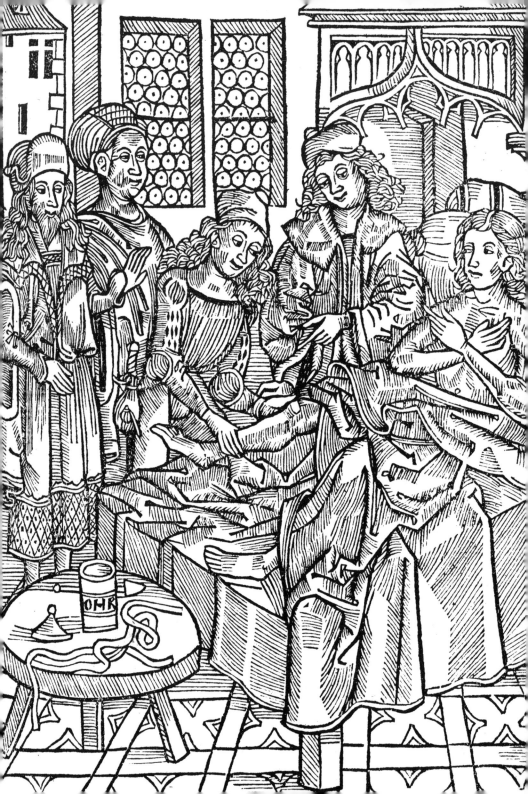

How to Cure the *Plague*
& Other Curious Remedies

JULIAN WALKER

THE BRITISH LIBRARY

First published in 2013 by
The British Library
96 Euston Road
London NW1 2DB

Cataloguing in publication data
A catalogue record for this book is available from the British Library

ISBN 978 0 7123 5701 2

Designed and typeset in Monotype Garamond by illuminati, Grosmont
Printed in Hong Kong by Great Wall Printing Co. Ltd

CONTENTS

INTRODUCTION

DISCUSSIONS based on the question 'which period of history would you most like to have lived in?' founder as soon as we consider the subject of medicine; we scurry back to the safety of modern hospitals, surgeries and doctors. But was medicine in the distant past so different, so bizarre and distressing? Did people, until the late Victorian era, live in a dark age of blood-letting, wilful ignorance of hygiene and the ingestion of medicines made from powdered toads and brandy?

Yes and no. Certainly, looking at pre-modern medical procedures can be frustrating at times – straightforward procedures such as washing hands and boiling water would have saved many lives; yet for thousands of years people have been using simple, natural ingredients in medicines that worked then, and still work now. The truth is that while many remedies from the past were absurd, misguided and horrific, many were viable; they can provoke recognition as well as horror, amazement and amusement.

Early medieval healing in England was largely based on observation of the effects of herbs and the use of prayer; some classical learning survived, and a few drugs and recipes from the eastern Mediterranean were in use. But from the twelfth century the reappearance in southern Italy of texts by Hippocrates, Galen, Dioscorides and Aristotle changed the course of European medicine. These texts, many of them preserved in the Arabic-language writings of the scholar known in Europe as Avicenna, were disseminated from the medical schools at Salerno and Montpellier, and later at Bologna, Paris, Padua and Oxford. A seven-year university degree included the study of Galen, Dioscorides' work on the medical use of herbs, and Aristotle's systematic observation of nature, together with some dietetics and observation of a human dissection.

Galen, a Roman doctor living in the second century AD, developed the ideas of the Greek physician Hippocrates (*c.* 460–370 BC), in which the body was governed by 'humours', which had to be kept balanced. The four humours were blood, yellow bile, black bile and phlegm; an excess of any one of these tilted the individual's temperament in one direction. Thus an excess of blood produced a sanguine temperament, yellow bile a choleric temperament, black bile a melancholic temperament and phlegm a phlegmatic (calm) temperament. Thinking of these humours as the four points of a compass, between blood and yellow bile lay the idea of heat, between yellow and black bile lay dryness, between black bile and phlegm lay coldness, and between phlegm and blood lay wetness. The theory of humours governed moods, medicines, ingredients, raw foods and cooking methods. Alchemy was involved through the various preparations of 'simples' – the untreated raw ingredients – using distillation, decoction (extraction through boiling) and so on. This complex system governed how most people thought about the body, illness and health until well into the seventeenth century.

An essential treatment in pre-modern medicine was bleeding and cupping (provoking the flow of blood by placing heated glass cups on broken skin); it was thought not only to effect a cure by taking blood away where there was an excess, but also to act as a preventive by removing excesses of humours, and especially removing so-called evil humours:

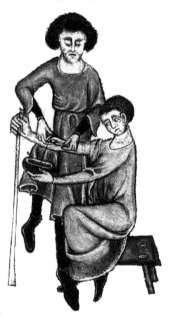

> Blood-letting in measure cleareth thy thought,
> it closeth thy bladder, it tempereth thy brain, it
> amendeth thy hearing, it strengtheneth tears,
> it closeth thy stomach, it digesteth thy food, it
> cleareth thy voice, it sharpeneth thy wit, it easeth
> thy womb, it bringeth on sleep, it draweth away
> anguish, it nourisheth good blood, it destroyeth
> wicked blood, and lengtheneth thy life.
>
> *Rosa Medicinae*, John of Gaddesden,
> fourteenth century

Plasters (effectively poultices) were used in the same way, to encourage or discourage heat or moisture and so balance the humours. Blistering plasters irritated the skin and drew pus – seen as poisonous matter – to the surface, where it could be removed.

One of the longest-lasting obsessions in British medicine was the idea of 'purging the system'. This meant either provoking vomit, or more often emptying the bowels. In the fourteenth century John of Ardenne was an enthusiastic proponent of enemas, both for cleansing and nourishing, and the idea of 'regularity' became part of a moral system as well as a physical regimen:

> One thing more there is, which has a great influence upon the health, and that it is, *going to stool* regularly. People that are very *loose*, have seldom strong thoughts, or strong bodies; but the cure of this, both by diet and medicine, being much more easie than the contrary evil, there needs not much to be said about it.
>
> *Some Thoughts Concerning Education*, John Locke, 1693

Using these methods the humours could be rebalanced, and more or less any disease resolved. *The Treasury of Hidden Secrets* (1659) proposed a recipe that was: 'A perfect way to cure the loathsome disease of the French pox, pains in the loins, lameness of limbs, paleness of colour, loathsome scabbes, or any other filthy disease proceeding of superfluous or evil humours; as also to assuage over-grosse and foggie fat bellies; and that without danger.'

Galen's system of humours was challenged in the sixteenth century by Paracelsus, a Swiss physician who believed that experience, rather than belief in authorities, would provide the answers to medical problems. While maintaining a belief in the occult, he encouraged the use of minerals, especially salt, mercury and sulphur, and a perception of disease as invading the body. After Paracelsus physicians gradually lost faith in authoritative texts, and there was a move towards a truly empirical chemistry in the service of healing.

Paracelsus was a great believer in the doctrine of signatures. This proposed that for every disease there was an antidote residing in something that a benign deity had placed on earth. All humans had to do was find, interpret and apply the correct herb, mineral or animal part or extract. It would be known because it looked like a symptom of the disease, or had some clear connection. Thus pulmonaria (lungwort) leaves looked like lungs, so people inferred that the plant was intended as a treatment for lung diseases. Sometimes these interpretations seem to be stretching the point, to modern eyes: a purple rash, for example, could be cured by eating purple silk washed down with ale.

Most early books of recipes and remedies include at least one medicine that promises to cure everything, or at least to fully cure one malady, and occasionally medicines offered tantalizing promises. The despair attendant upon syphilis was temporarily – but only temporarily – dispelled by the internal or external application of mercury, which has antiseptic qualities; long-term the disease would reappear. However, because mercury seemed able to treat such a painful and 'unfair' condition, its apparently benign qualities acquired a kind of mythical status: William Salmon in his edition of *Bates' Dispensatory* (1694) wrote that a mercury-based recipe ascribed to Paracelsus 'cures not only the French Pox, with all its attendants, and the dropsy, but also the gout, scabs, and leprosy; this need not seem strange to them who know that mercury is the balsam of Nature, in which [there] is an incarnative and regenerative virtue, wonderfully renovative and restorative, and cleansing from all impurities.' One can sense the delight in the trust in something that actually worked against the power of disease.

In the later medieval period the authority assigned to the texts of Galen and Hippocrates led those who had studied them to assume the roles of licensing authorities, sometimes in conflict with town councils or guilds, who took a more relaxed view. In Britain, the Royal College of Physicians was set up in 1518 to regulate practice. Women, excluded from British universities till the nineteenth century, were officially excluded from most medical practice, but were licensed as midwives and practitioners in the treatment of women and children; and women's first-hand knowledge of such things as diet and childcare meant that

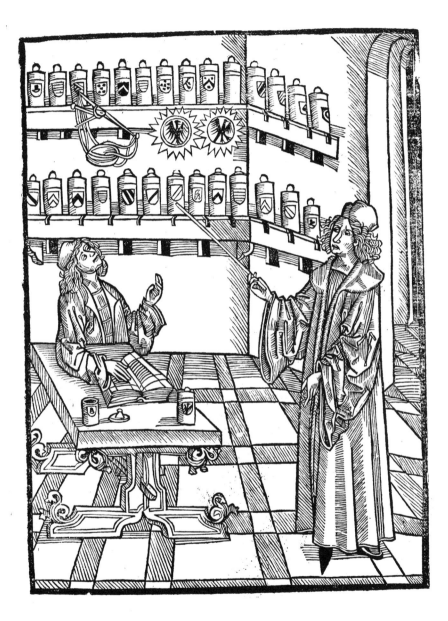

they were often the first people consulted in the case of disease. Barber-surgeons had been responsible for what happened on the outside of the body (and in instances when, through trauma, the inside became the outside), while the higher-status physicians dealt with what went on inside. This distinction broke down between 1500 and 1700, and many surgeons were grudgingly accepted by physicians, especially when conditions such as fistulas or piles responded only to surgical treatment. Apothecaries, at first merchants in drugs and ingredients, became more than shopkeepers; the Society of Apothecaries, formed in 1617, was legally authorized to prescribe medicines a hundred years later, though it was shadowed by legions of unregulated chemists and quacks.

The clear distinctions between surgeons, physicians and apothecaries did not always work in the patient's favour. It was perhaps the too-rigid following of theories that led practitioners up blind alleys, from which their prestige and incomes disinclined them to emerge. It was also all too easy for the patient to feel that some deal was going on between the physician and the apothecary. Nicholas Culpeper, writing in the mid-seventeenth century, made recommendations to avoid paying apothecaries for plants that could be gathered freely, while Gideon Harvey in *The Family-Physician and the House-Apothecary* (1676) wrote that 'in preparing medicines thus at your own houses … it's not only a far safer way, but that you shall also save nineteen shillings in twenty, comparing it with the extravagant rates of many apothecaries'.

Culpeper saw it as his mission to encourage people to practise medicine without having recourse to the controlling busybodies at the Royal College of Physicians, or the apothecaries, whom he felt were out to make money from trusting and desperate invalids. In his translation from Latin into English of the *Dispensatory* of the 'Colledge of Physitians of London' (1651) he complained that the writers confused their information and did not fully know the meanings of the words they used.

As medicine was a commercial commodity, competition among practitioners involved disparaging rival medicines; an Almanack for 1747 stated the following:

For your distilled waters, the greatest number of them are as cordial as water stagnated in a ditch. They are vapid and apalling to the taste. The blood and spirits will be better pleased and strengthened with the infusion of those herbs, though it be in fountain water, and much preferable to any kind of syrup; for all syrups are clogging, windy in the stomach, and fermentative in the bowels.

The increasingly important scientific process of the observation of symptoms led to the identification of major diseases, but present-day and historical terms do not always correlate: we cannot be absolutely sure what a sixteenth-century physician meant when he referred to the 'flux' or a 'noli me tangere'. Many terms for diseases, treatments and ingredients have dropped out of use, while some recognizable ones have lost their original meanings or gained new ones: 'distillation' was used to describe not just the process of boiling a mixture to obtain a purified liquid by condensation of vapour, but also for ramming a paste into an upended flask and collecting the liquid that oozed out.

There is one disease that stands out from the rest, immediately recognizable and deeply feared. William Salmon's translation of *Bates' Dispensatory* (1694) contained this description of cordials (heart stimulant): 'Cordials defend the Heart and Vitals against all manner of Infection of the Measles, Small and Pox, Purples, Spotted Feaver, or any other Malign Feaver; yea, and against the Plague itself.'

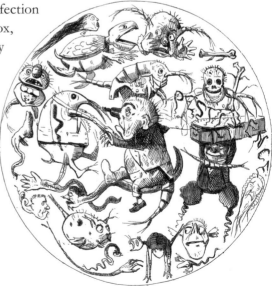

This quote shows how much the plague was feared as the most pestilential of all epidemics, with clear signs of its inevitable resolution as the flesh turned black and died. In *A Most Excellent and Perfect Homish Apothecarye*

(1561), John Hollybush's translation of Hieronymus Braunschweig's book, we read 'It is to be remarked that when he that hath the pestilence bleedeth and cannot be staunched nor cease, it is an evident and sure sign of death.' Though smallpox killed more people, the plague was instantly and terrifyingly recognizable, with black eruptions and boils, and often death within a day.

Between 1600 and 1800 a variety of approaches to medicine coexisted, including folk medicine, academic 'physick' and common sense. The gradual increase in the use of scientific observations and the growth of respect for surgeons in the eighteenth century did not dispel the widespread use of cupping and bleeding, though the Galenic system of humours fell out of use. Some old theories died hard; the idea of 'poisoned air' persisted into the nineteenth century.

In cities increased population density largely cancelled out the improvements in medicine until a direct link was made between public sanitation and disease – in 1854 Dr John Snow stopped an epidemic of cholera by removing the handle of the infected water pump in Broad Street in Soho, London. Germ theory discredited the idea of infected air, and with anaesthesia it was no longer necessary to perform operations at breakneck speed. The nineteenth century saw changes in medicine that dispelled most of the myths and horrors of early-modern disease and treatment.

It should not be assumed, however, that before the major breakthroughs of the nineteenth century all medicine was unsound; still less that the further back in time we look the more unsound it was. For example, smoky houses, dirty towns and dense living conditions have all contributed throughout history to eye infections as a common hazard of life in the British Isles. Diagnoses in *Bald's Leechbook* (*c.*950) describe 'misty eyes', 'eye pain', cataracts, 'eye-shrinkage', 'worms in the eyes' and what seem to be trachoma and xerophthalmia. But looking at the large number of treatments for eye conditions, dating back to the earliest medical texts written in Old English, we can see that some of them are sound and viable, based on observation and experience.

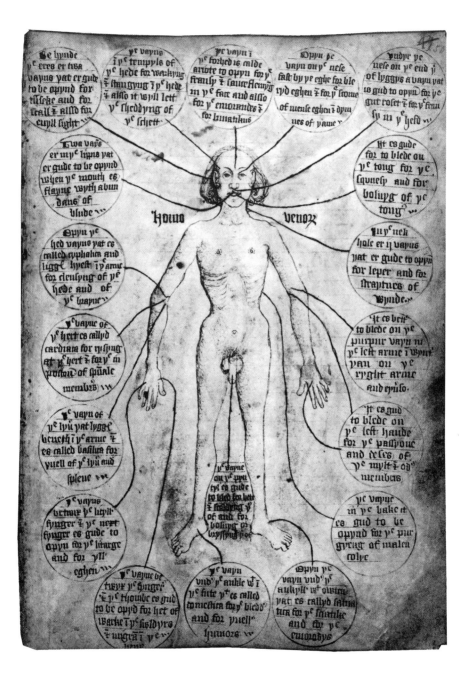

A twelfth-century text, the *Peri Didaxeon*, recommends for poor night vision 'roasted buck-liver, from which a liquid flows out when it is roasted; anoint the eyes with it and give the liver itself to be eaten.' Liver is indeed rich in Vitamin A, which is beneficial to the eyes.

Early medical texts show some major diseases such as leprosy that have now largely disappeared, and also show that the threats to health have changed. In past eras different kinds of disease or trauma predominated. In the seventeenth and eighteenth centuries 'the stone' (in the bladder or kidneys) concerned people, gout and dropsy were widespread and there were many possible treatments for the bites of venomous snakes and mad dogs. These reflect the changing social conditions, the availability, quality and prices of sweet foods or other comestibles, and surges in public concern.

So how different an experience of medicine do we have from our ancestors 300, 500 or 800 years ago? For them there was a range of maladies that physicians optimistically claimed to be able to resolve through the use of particular medicines or treatments; these might range from melancholy to gout, taking in leprosy and epilepsy. But is such a blanket approach any more worrying than the range of potential side-effects listed for the majority of modern prescription medicines? Do we not choose for the most part to ignore these, just as the seventeenth-century invalid focused on the one ailment he or she needed to be cured of?

Just as William Langham swore by rhubarb in the sixteenth century and William Buchan praised blood-letting in the eighteenth, we now have our individual medical talismans; our preferred brands of painkiller or stomach-settler. Our eighteenth-century forebears were as dependent on proprietary medicines as we are. Like Gideon Harvey we know that medicines are far more expensive than they need to be, and even after thousands of years of experience and trial and error most of us are still not entirely sure how to deal with a splinter or a nosebleed.

Over the past hundred years medicine has changed fundamentally, but just how different are today's patients from those who queued at the medieval monastery door, or 300 years ago looked up the right combination of herbs to soothe an ague?

This book is organized along the lines of how we see our bodies and named maladies when we are sick. Illness makes us concentrate on the affected parts, while major maladies like 'jaundice' or 'smallpox' largely remain as separate, abstract ideas. A book of remedies creates a kind of virtual patient, a recipient of treatments directed at different parts, but brought together in one place. So this book may be thought of as a lifetime's experience of disease and medicine, with illnesses, diagnoses and treatments that are by turn bewildering, plausible, bizarre and touching. Above all it shows the twists and turns, and the occasional direct routes, that people have taken in the business of trying to understand the processes of disease and the restoration of health. Between 1850 and 1950 the introduction of anaesthesia and antibiotics, the acceptance of germ theory, the awareness of vitamins and so on, brought the practice of medicine into being something we are generally content to accept today; this book stops where the recipes and remedies that were orthodox medicine start to become curious and questionable.

The texts use come from a range of publications, handbills, pamphlets, medical textbooks and domestic compendia. Some of them were ephemeral, while some remained in print for many years: *Gerard's Herbal* is still in print over four centuries after it first appeared, while William Buchan's *Domestic Medicine* ran to over twenty editions. Texts such as these often would have been one of only three or four books owned by a working family.

Primarily I have selected texts which put into words people's experience of medicine – the recipes describe what they would receive in terms of medication and treatment. For that reason I have tried to retain something of the flavour of the English used at different periods, while making it as readable as possible to the modern layperson. I have changed as little as possible, but changes include modernizing spellings, translation where necessary, and simplifying some of the near-impenetrable language of the apothecaries.

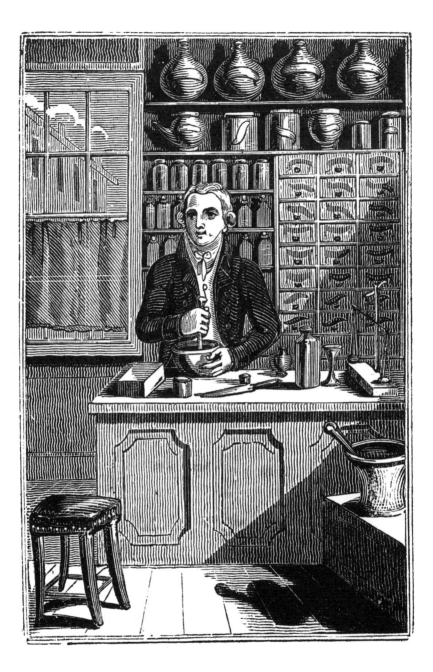

Heart, liver and lights

WHILE the function and importance of the heart and the lungs were established early on, the role of the liver was less clear. Francis Bacon, in his book *A Natural History in Ten Centuries* (1627), wrote of 'the operation of the liver, in sending down the wheyey part of the blood to the reins [kidneys]'.

Wintergreen

The herb boiled in wine and water and given to drink to them that have any inward ulcers in their kidneys or neck of the bladder, doth wonderfully help them; it stayeth also all fluxes, whether of blood or humours, [such] as the lask, bloody flux, women's courses, and bleeding of the womb, and taketh away any inflammation rising upon pains of the heart.

The English Physitian, Nicholas Culpeper, 1652

☞ Oil of wintergreen, now obtained by distillation of the leaves, contains methyl salicylate, similar to aspirin, which is a longstanding treatment for cardiovascular conditions including heart attacks, acting as an anti-inflammatory and blood thinner.

A good medicine for the passion of the Heart

Take red rose leaves, oil of mace, and powder of saffron, and mingle them all together, and quilt them in a little thin silk, and draw it over with a little thin civet, and so apply it to the region of the heart, and it will do you marvellous much good.

A Rich Storehouse, or Treasurie for the Diseased, 1607

☞ This elegant dry plaster seems to have been perfumed with civet, a musk-like fragrance from the animal of the same name, that was extremely expensive. A 'passion' here meant any painful disorder.

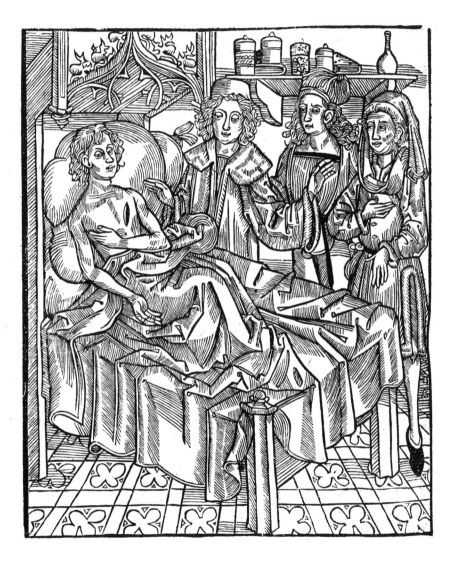

Of hearte's feebleness or faintness

That cometh thereby when the filth is so increased about [the heart], that it can not expel and cast it from it. This filth is engendered by great surfeiting and excess specially in such [people] as surfeit & labour not, whereby their stomach waxeth so full that it can not digest. Or else if a man had eaten meat evil to digest, whereby the body is filled with overmuch wind & the heart enfeebled, whereof man getteth many diseases and inconveniences, [such] as scabbes, yushes, or wheales, mattering sores, karnels and the canker.

It is to be noted that nothing is better for a faintness of hearte, than that a man put whole saffron in his drink, and put always a little in his broth or potage: that comforteth the hearte very well & warmeth a man.

A Most Excellent and Perfect Homish Apothecarye, John Hollybush's translation of Hieronymus Braunschweig, 1561

☛ The high cost of saffron would have made this remedy plausible only for the very rich. Saffron is supposed to be good for the blood, but toxic to the nervous system above a certain – fortunately prohibitively expensive – level. There is a noteworthy association here between heart disease, overeating and lack of exercise. 'Mattering sores' were ones that produced matter – effectively pus; 'karnels' were inflamed swellings; 'yushes' seems to be a typesetter's mistake, and should have been 'pushes' – boils.

Heartache

For the cardiache and swelling at the heart, make a drink of rosemary with rosewater or white wine; or else a syrup with rosewater or white wine, with the juice of parsnips, sugar, and the bone of a stag's heart, and use thereof.

To comfort the heart, seethe rosemary, and the flowers with rosewater, and drink it.

The Garden of Health, William Langham, 1578

🖛 Deer do indeed have a bone in the heart, which in the early-modern world fascinated people; it became endowed with medicinal properties. Rosemary is noted as being beneficial to a heart subject to palpitations.

For the liver

From the liver of a man will be drawn by distillation a water and an oil. If the water be drunk every morning together, by the space of a month, in the quantity of one dram, with two ounces of liverwort, it will recover such as are half rotten through diseases of the liver; and it hath divers other properties.

Polypharmakos, Daniel Border, 1651

🖛 The use of the human body itself as a source of raw materials for medicines is one of the little-known stories of European medicine. It is not quite cannibalism, though it is only the process of what is in effect alchemy that makes such a description avoidable.

For a hard liver

Liver hard, apply a plaster of dwale and raisins.

The Garden of Health, William Langham, 1578

🖛 'Dwale' was a painkiller; in some cases an infusion of belladonna (deadly nightshade), but also sometimes including lettuce, bryony, henbane or opium. Several conditions could cause pain in the liver, but cirrhosis would cause the liver to shrink and become 'hard'.

Asthma

Live a fortnight on boiled carrots only. It seldom fails.

Primitive Physick, John Wesley, 1755

🖛 Wesley proposed a return to a system that supposedly existed before physicians exerted control over the world of medicine, when people used common materials. This remedy required some commitment from the patient, who would possibly have begun to change colour by the end of it (yellow rather than orange, from hypercarotenemia).

A drink against lung disease

Boil horehound in wine or ale, sweeten slightly with honey; give it to drink warm having fasted for a night, and then let him lie on his right side for a good while after the drinking and stretch out his right arm as far as he can.

The Lacnunga, eleventh century

↘ Horehound has for millennia been used in treatments for coughs and lung complaints; the first-century Greek physician Dioscorides recommended it as a remedy for shortness of breath. Here it is combined with a description of what may be the Anglo-Saxon recovery position.

Breathing troubles

The pulp of the middle ribs of colewort boiled in almond milk, and made up into an electuary with honey, being taken often, is very profitable for those that are pursic and short-winded. Being boiled twice, and an old cock boiled in the broth and drunk, it helpeth the pains and obstructions in the liver and spleen, and the stone in the kidneys.

The English Physitian, Nicholas Culpeper, 1652

↘ 'Colewort' was the name given to several plants of the cabbage family. If you were 'pursic' you had difficulty breathing.

A marvellous good medicine to preserve the lungs

Take the lungs of a fox and dry it well, and beat it to a powder, and then put a quarter of a spoonful thereof into a little new almond milk, or else into some other thin broth made of veal or mutton, and let the patient eat it, and this will preserve the lungs wonderfully greatly.

A Rich Storehouse, or Treasurie for the Diseased, 1607

☞ Did people using this direct approach (matching the cure very literally to the ailment) take some symbolic strength from a particular animal – and if so, why a fox? Perhaps it had to do with the availability of a free and lively animal that could be caught legally.

Sighing

The powder of the root of elecampane mixed with sugar and honey is a blessed medicine against shortness of breath, sighing and coughing; it cleanseth the breast and healeth the impostumes of the lungs, matrix and other parts or entrails.

The Garden of Health, William Langham, 1578

☞ The 'matrix' here is the womb. Elecampane is a rich source of inulin, a polysaccharide that promotes the absorption of calcium and the growth of intestinal bacteria. It has long been used in the treatment of lung disorders.

Asthmatic emulsion

Take millipedes, about 120, bruise them in a mortar, pouring on them by little and little pennyroyal water, six ounces, dissolve in it gum ammoniac, three drams; strain it and take a table spoonful once a day in a cup of marshmallow or colt's foot tea.

All asthmatic persons should have a seton or issue, set in the arm or thigh, which would have an excellent effect.

Plaster for the asthma – take burgundy pitch; if it is too hard mix a little turpentine or olive oil (that it may stick to the part for some time), apply it between the shoulders and when it gets moist take it off, wipe it and put it on again.

The Family Physician, Edward Bullman, 1789

☞ Burgundy pitch is the resinous gum of the spruce-fir, which was believed to draw moisture from the chest. Some species of millipedes, when threatened, release a toxin that may be narcotic, but there is no reason why this should provide any relief for asthma. The 'millipedes' may in this case be woodlice, also known as millipedes or sows at that time.

A 'seton' – a cloth soaked in medicine – when inserted into a cut performed a function similar to that of an injection, introducing *materia medica* into the bloodstream, but presumably with some degree of pain and a high risk of infection.

A receipt for the pleurisy

Take three round balls of horse-dung, boil them in a pint of white wine till half be consumed, then strain it out and sweeten it with a little sugar, and let the patient go to bed and drink this, then lay him warm.

A choice manual of rare and select secrets in physick and chyrurgery, Elizabeth Grey, 1653

☞ It is difficult to know how this could have done any good at all. Hopefully the extended boiling period may have destroyed some of the pathogens in the dung.

Elizabeth Grey was Countess of Kent, and this collection of recipes was collated for her use and published after her death, rather than written by her.

FIRE DOWN BELOW

I N THE DAYS before hygienic sanitation, medical problems located in the private parts must have rendered invalids absolutely wretched. We can only admire the energy with which people ranged in the search for treatments for such miserable conditions.

For the piles

Take one spoonful of white dogs turd, as much white frankincense, and twenty four grains of aloes, beat them fine and searce [sift] them, then take one spoonful of honey, the yolk of an egg, and as much oil of roses as will make it an ointment, mingle them well together and anoint the grieved place; if the sore be inward, wet a tent of lint in the ointment and put it in the fundament, and spread some of the ointment on a cloth, and put that on it. This is a present remedy.

The Queens Closet Opened, W.M., 1696

☞ 'Present' here means 'fast-acting', while a 'tent' was a soft cloth or plaster used to keep a sore open. The application of dog excrement shocks modern sensibilities, but the material was much used in early-modern times, especially in tanning, in which it was called 'pure'. The following page of *The Queens Closet Opened* carried a remedy for a sore throat, with ingredients including egg yolk, honey and 'white dogs turd', but the making process and application are probably best consigned to history.

For the swelling of the yard or cods

Take agrimony, of the water thereof distilled, and put thereto a quantity of alum, and set them over the fire till they almost boil: then with a rag of linen cloth anoint the yard under the skin with the water well and warm: and it will abate the pain of the yard and of the cods also, if they be washed with the same. And to incarnate the skin of the yard within, take the water of fumitory, and lay liquorice pared therein one night, and put of the same water into the yard with a sponge, or else with a tent of linen cloth.

The Widdowes Treasure, 1639

☙ To 'incarnate' meant to cause flesh to grow, or to heal. The 'cods' and 'yard' were the male genitals (hence the word 'codpiece'). Alum is an astringent and styptic, and speeds the healing of sores and wounds, so might have helped reduce inflammation. Fumitory is a herb traditionally valued for its purifying power.

Distillation would have been carried out at home: 'Every young gentlewoman is to be furnished with very good stills, for the distillation of all kind of waters; which stills must be either of tin, or fine earthenware, and in them she shall distill all manner of waters, meet for the health of her household.' *The Ladies Dictionary* (1694)

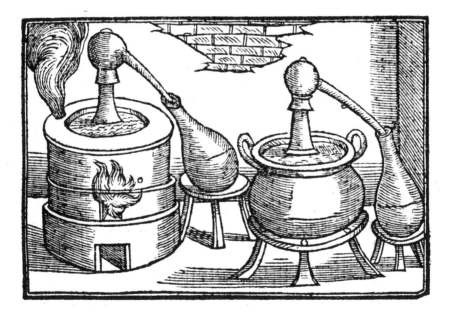

Of the pain of the hemorrhoids

The sick person is tormented with a most intense pain, when he voideth excrements, the surface of which is also sprinkled with blood. Sometimes tumours like warts lurk inwardly in the muscle called the sphincter, or appear in the brims of the fundament.

Let ten ounces of blood be taken out of the right arm.

Take of frogs sperm water, four ounces; dissolve in it of litharge, two drams: opium one scruple. Apply a linen clout soaked in a little of this mixture to the part affected; or if the tumour lurk inwardly, inject three spoonfuls of the same mixture by way of a clyster.

The Compleat Method of Curing Almost All Diseases,
Thomas Sydenham, 1694

🐟 'Frogs sperm water' (probably frogspawn) is a surprising ingredient to modern readers, but in a pre-industrial age the natural world – any part of it – was an immediate source of *materia medica*. Litharge was a lead oxide. Thomas Sydenham, known as 'the father of English medicine' and 'the English Hippocrates', in the seventeenth century regularly recommended fresh air and exercise as a treatment, and popularized a tincture of opium (laudanum), which was used, probably excessively, as an effective painkiller over the next 150 years. Apothecaries' weights were as follows: 1 ounce = 8 drams/drachms = 24 scruples = 480 grains.

Swelling in the generative parts

First the patient should be bled in the arm, or leeches may be applied to the inflamed parts; afterwards take a handful of green rue, bruise it, and put it to the part affected; or take marshmallows a handful, camomile a handful, make a decoction in a pint of water, pour the liquor from the herbs, add two drams of the tincture of opium, bathe the part; afterwards apply the herbs as a poultice, or make a poultice of oatmeal and vinegar with a little sweet oil in it. Warts and chancres may be destroyed, by touching the warts with a blue stone vitriol, or ... by washing them with a solution of corrosive sublimate.

The Family Physician, Edward Bullman, 1789

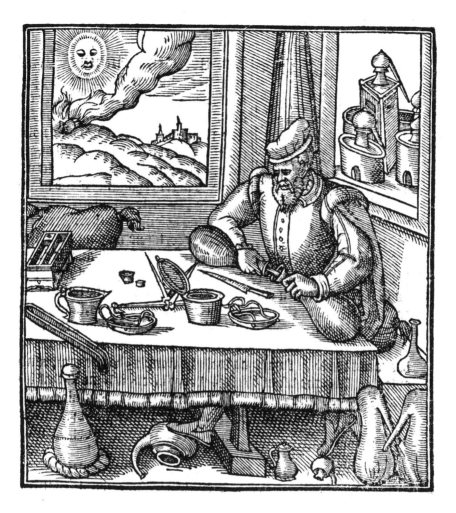

☞ 'Blue stone vitriol' was a solution of copper sulphate, effective as an antiseptic, but it can burn skin, especially in sensitive areas. Whether it would be preferable to leeches in this case is a difficult call. And 'a solution of corrosive sublimate' was mercuric chloride; when you thought things couldn't get any worse, you'll be pleased to know this was formerly used to burn away corns.

Toothache

The teeth are created to chew the meat therewith that it may be the more apt to digestion, they aid also to the speech, to retain the breth and to man's adorning and continence. They have also pain and smart, as other members or limbs, namely gnawing, holes, wormes, wagging, apostumation in the gums, corrupt humors and blood of the gums.

A Most Excellent and Perfect Homish Apothecarye, John Hollybush's
translation of Hieronymus Braunschweig, 1561

For the teeth

If you will keep your teeth from rotting or aching, wash the mouth continually every morning with juice of lemons, and afterwards rub your teeth with a sage leaf, and wash your teeth after meat with fair water.

To cure the tooth ache:

Take mastic and chew it in your mouth till it is as soft as wax, then stop your teeth with it, if hollow, there remaining till it is consumed, and it will certainly cure you.

The tooth of a dead man carried about a man, presently suppresses the pains of teeth.

The Queens Closet Opened,
W.M., 1696

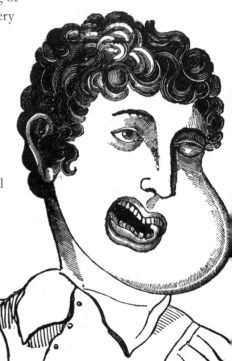

☛ The stopping of a hole, which the tongue would be aware of, is a sensible approach compared to the magic of the tooth-amulet.

To make a tooth to fall without smart

The gray worms breathing under wood or stones having many feet, and when they be touched do they cluster together like porkenpickes [porcupines]; these pierced through with a bodkin or like thing and then put into the tooth that acheth allayeth the pain. Like wise doth also a little slice of the root of alcorus, of some called in English gladdon, of other galanga [galingale], which groweth in waters and marasses; this must be laid green upon the tooth. A piece of the green root of tormentil doth likewise.

A Most Excellent and Perfect Homish Apothecarye, John Hollybush's translation of Hieronymus Braunschweig, 1561

☛ Curiously gladdon, or sweet flag (*Acorus calamus*), has insecticidal properties, which would be useful if toothache were actually caused by worms in the teeth. The root of tormentil (the name is applied to both cranesbill and cinquefoil) is good for mouth sores. Putting a woodlouse against a decayed tooth is an interesting idea; as affordable dentists become increasingly scarce, remedies like this may be useful to know.

An approved remedy for the toothache

The roots of henbane sodden in vinegar and rosewater; put the decocotion in your mouth.

The Widdowes Treasure, 1639

☛ Don't; the whole plant is poisonous. John Gerard in his famous *History of Plants* (1597) stated that 'mountebank tooth-drawers' would burn the seeds of henbane in a dish, holding the toothache-sufferer's head over the smoke, and then pretending to find worms in the patient's mouth. The 'worms' would in fact be fragments of lute string.

WARTS AND ALL

W ARTS have puzzled people for millennia. Their appearance and (sometimes) mystifying sudden disappearance have provoked some of the most bewildering recipes.

An Anglo-Saxon treatment for warts

For warts take hound's urine and mouse's blood, mixed together, anoint the warts with it, they will soon go away.

Leechdom (Anglo-Saxon manuscript)

☛ The source of the ingredients being the smallest and largest animals to be found in a domestic space may be important, though urine has traditionally been used for styptic purposes.

For an anthrax

If peacocks' droppings be applied, it breaks, ripens, and heals the anthrax. Bruise daisies between two stones, and put them on it, and raw yolks of eggs, and burnt salt, mixed well, and this will break it by the end of the third day.

Rosa Medicinae, John of Gaddesden, fourteenth century

☛ Until the nineteenth century 'an anthrax' was a boil or carbuncle.

An alexiterien mummy of life

[This] is the blood of a lusty and healthful man dried with a gentle fire, impregnated with the spirit of lemons, and spirit of vitriol, and a little myrrh made into trochisces.

It is very efficacious in curing carbuncles.

The History of Animals as They are Useful in Physick and Chirurgery, John Schroder, 1659

🖙 'Alexiteriens' (or alexiterians) were medicines taken against poison; 'trochisces' were tablets. The widespread early-modern practice of taking human blood as a rejuvenating practice may at first seem horrific, but research at Stanford University publicized in 2012 shows that this works on mice, and may have rejuvenating applications on humans.

Turnsole or heliotropum

The seed and juice of the leaves being rubbed with a little salt upon warts, wens, and other hard kernels in the face, eyelids, or any other part of the body, will by often using take them away.

The English Physitian, Nicholas Culpeper, 1652

🖙 Heliotrope and turnsole were names given to various plants which turned to face the sun; if this recipe used valerian, which is heliotropic, it would have been effective against skin disorders, as that plant has antibacterial properties.

Shingles

The patients took for them doves' dung newly made; and barley meal; stamped them well, and mixed them with half a pint of vinegar; they used it cold to the place grieved and applied vine leaves (to keep in the liquor) round about it, then they bound it up with clothes and suffered it to lie three days and then (if need were) refreshed it again with a new plaster, and at the most with the use of these applications, it was perfectly helped.

Polypharmakos, Daniel Border, 1651

☞ Wet barley meal, with a high starch content and kept moist on the skin, would have provided some relief to shingles sufferers. Doves' dung, however new, is not recommended.

Headlice

For the lice of the head take a pennyworth of laurel or bay berries, bray them to powder; tie them in a linen cloth; seethe the same in running water and wash the head therewith. The same virtue hath also the root of bearfoot beaten to powder.

A Most Excellent and Perfect Homish Apothecarye,
John Hollybush's translation of Hieronymus Braunschweig, 1561

☞ Laurel leaves contain prussic acid, traditionally used by collectors to kill butterflies and moths; the berries of laurel are toxic. 'Bearfoot' was an alternative name for black hellebore and monkshood, both of which are toxic and irritate the skin.

A great wen taken away

One that was troubled with a great wen had it taken away, by washing it with a strong lye made of skin ashes. I have been told since of a certain, that if ye rub the wen often with the hand of a dead man until the wen wax hot it will consume away in a short time after. Some roast an egg hard, and cut it in the midst, and lay it thereon, and using this often the wen will wear away.

Polypharmakos, Daniel Border, 1651

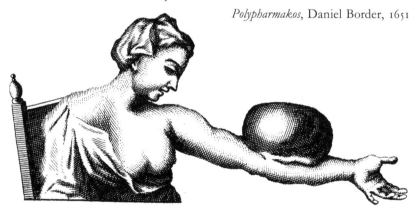

The mysterious appearance of a 'wen' (defined by Thomas Churchill as 'a tumour or excrescence, consisting of a bag filled with some peculiar matter'), and its often equally mysterious disappearance, must have confused people and provoked all kinds of attempts to control the manifestation. During this period of history 'the hand of a dead man' would have been more accessible than at present. The traditional treatment in the early twentieth century was to hit the wen unexpectedly with a copy of Grey's *Anatomy*, the huge anatomical authority, with some doctors believing that this was the book's most useful role in the surgery.

To take away warts

Take snails that have shells, pick them, and with the juice that cometh from them rub the wart every day for the space of seven or eight days, and it will destroy them.

A Choice Manual of Rare and Select Secrets in Physick and Chyrurgery, Elizabeth Grey, 1653

While snail mucus is used in various parts of the world for medical and cosmetic purposes, the scientific community is still divided as to its efficacy. The visual similarity between warts and snail shells and toad skin has inevitably led to those animals' unwilling participation in treatment.

Dandruff

The juice of the mallows boiled in old oil and applied, [and] the decocotion of beets in water and some vinegar healeth the itch, if bathed therewith, and cleanseth the head of dandruff, scurf, and dry scabs, and doth much good for fretting and running sores, ulcers, & cankers in the head, legs, or other parts, and is much commended against baldness and shedding of hair.

The juice, or distilled water of the herb is effectual for green wounds, or old sores, and cleanseth the body inwardly; and the seed outwardly, from sores, scurf, itches, pimples, freckles, morphew, or other deformities thereof, but especially if a little vitriol be dissolved therein.

The English Physitian, Nicholas Culpeper, 1652

≈ Taken internally and externally, the common mallow and marsh mallow have several healing properties; gum and starch, together with salicylic acid, render the plant useful for treating skin ailments. Antioxidants in beet also benefit the skin. 'Green wounds' were fresh wounds, and a 'morphew' was any discoloration of the skin caused by disease.

An eruption

Against a burst eruption: take a swallow's nest and break it up wholly, and burn it wholly with dung, and crumble it to dust, and mix with vinegar and smear with it.

The Lacnunga, eleventh century

≈ Chinese medicine regards the swallow's nest, containing calcium, iron, potassium, magnesium and protein, as having a beneficial effect on the skin and lungs. Mixing it with dung and burning it would not be likely to enhance any of its virtues.

Galling and excoriation

These are very troublesome to children. They happen chiefly about the groin and wrinkles of the neck, under the arms, behind the ears, and in other parts that are moistened by sweat or urine.

As these complaints are, in a great measure, owing to want of cleanliness, the most effectual means of preventing them are to wash the parts frequently with cold water, to change the linen often, and in a word, to keep the child, in all respects, thoroughly clean. When this is not sufficient, the excoriated parts may be sprinkled with absorbent or drying powders, [such] as burnt hartshorn, tutty, chalk, crabs claws prepared, and the like. When the parts affected are very sore, and tend to a real ulceration, it will be proper to add a little sugar of lead to the powders; or to anoint the place with the camphorated ointment. If the part be washed with spring-water, in which a little white vitriol has been dissolved, it will dry and heal them very powerfully. One of the best applications for this purpose, is to dissolve some fuller's earth in a sufficient quantity of hot water; and after it has stood till it is cold, to rub gently upon the galled parts once or twice a day.

Domestic Medicine, William Buchan, 1774

☞ The basic treatment for this rubbing of the skin has not changed much. 'Tutty' was a form of zinc oxide, which later came to be used in fabric plasters and is still a component of baby powders. 'Sugar of lead' (lead acetate) was used to sweeten wines, but is toxic when taken internally; as an emollient against skin irritation it has a long history, and until recently it was a component of treatments for grey hair and dandruff. 'White vitriol' (zinc sulphate), despite its rather worrying name, is widely used in treatments for skin disorders.

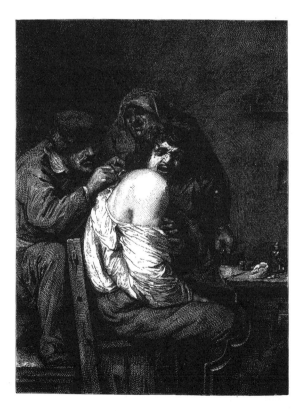

Ear, nose and throat

A sore throat, being a common early symptom of so many conditions, would have given weight to the idea of 'poisoned air'. One of the strongest-held beliefs of pre-modern medicine was that many diseases were caused by breathing 'bad air'; this is reflected in the word 'malaria'.

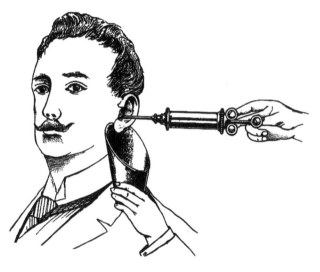

Earache

The smoke of tobacco blown into the ear, or a roasted onion or salt put into the ear, will take away the pain, but the head must be kept warm.

Every Patient His Own Doctor, Lewis Robinson, 1785

☞ Apparently hot salt applied to the ear can relieve pain, and anecdotal evidence indicates that the same effect can be had from tobacco smoke.

Two recipes for deafness

Mr Locher, an Apothecary of London, his excellent oil for deafness, which he gave to Sir Kenelm Digby; Another Experimented Remedy for the same

Take oil of bitter almonds, oil of spikenard, to each 6 drams; juice of onions, juice of rue, to each 2 drams; of black hellebore, colloquintada [bitter-apple, *Citrullus colocynthis*], oil of Exeter, 2 drams; boil this till the juice be consumed; then strain it, and add two drops of oil of aniseed, oil of origanum [oregano or marjoram] one drop. Pour a drop or two of this oil into the ear, and lie upon your bed with that ear upwards that you intend to drop into; lie still for a quarter of an hour after, then drop into the other, if it require. It is to be continued a month, or two or three, as you find benefit. When you have dropped into the ear, you must stop it with a little black-wool, dipped in the oil. Many persons have found much benefit by the use of this oil, to my knowledge.

Another Experimented Remedy for the same

Take a good large eel, flea it [skin it], and cut it into round pieces of the length of a finger, stick them full with rosemary and sage; then take an earthenware pan, put two or three sticks of wood in cross-wise, lay your pieces of eel upon them, so that they may not touch the bottom of the pan; bake it in an oven as you do meat; then take the fat of the eel that is in the pan, and strain it through a fine linen cloth, measure how much there is of it, and put to it as much spirits of wine. Then take juice of onions and juice of the white ends of leeks, to each one dram, [and] of your first mixture two drams; put them together into a vial, stop it close, and shake it well for an hour. It is in all things to be used as the former, except that instead of one or two drops you must drop in three or four.

Handbill, seventeenth century

🖘 In these seventeenth-century recipes the application of clarified oil to the ear as a treatment for thick wax is clearly recognizable; the second recipe begins alarmingly, but is basically animal fat with a little antibiotic onion juice.

Stoppage of the nose

Take hog's lard any quantity, mix a few drops of sweet oil with it, and rub the nostrils and between the eyes repeatedly till the mucus gets a free discharge; or the juice of a raw onion rubbed on the nose, between the eyes, will have the same effect.

The Family Physician, Edward Bullman, 1789

🖝 The absence of measurement for the lard allows for disconcerting images.

Of bleeding at the nose

Let the patient speak little, and let him eschew moving, trouble of mind, and chiefly anger. Also it is good to have the lower parts of the head highest. For the cure, you must take heed that in bleeding at the nose, the lower parts lie highest, and the head downward. The cure must be begun with those remedies which turn the blood to other parts of the body. First therefore if the body be full, and age will suffer it, and if the sick[ness] be not resolved, you must cut the veins on the arm, right against the flowing of the blood at the nose.

Moreover, friction and rubbing of the inferior parts, [such] as the arms, hands, thighs, share [groin], and feet is very profitable; and it is marvellously good to put the feet into warm water, ever rubbing them up and down.

The Method of Physick, Philip Barrough, 1639

🖝 Barrough's recommended treatment for a nosebleed develops into a whole-body experience involving cupping the liver area if the right nostril is bleeding, or the area of the spleen if the left nostril is bleeding; an ointment made from frankincense and 'the soft hairs of a hare' is applied to the nose, the ears are stopped 'strongly with linen and wax' and the patient should 'hold in the mouth cold rain water'. For good measure 'the flesh of snails brayed with vinegar, or their shells burnt and brayed' are good, and should be applied to the forehead as a paste, with vinegar.

If the bleeding has not stopped by then, and the patient is still within the grasp of whoever is treating him or her, the following treatment is to be deployed: 'above all the blood which cometh out of the patient's nose is good, if it be burned in an earthenware pot, and then beaten; take of it three drams, of bole-armoniac one scruple, of camphor one scruple, with the white of an egg and a little vinegar, make it thick like honey, and lay it to the forehead, and put it into the nose.'

In this case the last remedy in the list might work by frightening the patient into convincing him- or herself, and everyone else in the room, that recovery has been effected, and that the nosebleed has indeed stopped, even though there may be fountains of blood springing from the nostrils. 'Necessity requiring it, it is lawful to put too two grains or three of opium; asses' dung dried and made into a powder is wonderfully good, and also hogs' dung hath the like property.'

Another for nose-bleeds

In 1830 we were called in the night to see a man who had been for some time bleeding profusely at the nose; he was a poor labouring man, and had no fire in the house; the floor was literally covered with blood. We asked if he had met with an accident, or been in any way injured on the part. He answered that the bleeding had come on spontaneously; and the stream of blood then flowing from his nose was as thick as wheat-straw. We commenced operations by heating a little water in a tin can over the flame of a lamp, into which we put half a teaspoonful of cayenne pepper, and a teaspoonful of sugar. The patient held his nose, and drank the mixture, which had not been in his stomach more than a minute, before the bleeding stopped, although he could not have lost [less than] three quarts previously.

In this case there was a determination of blood to the head; but no sooner had the stomach felt the force of the stimulating pepper, than a reaction took place in the system, and the blood, instead of rushing to the head, was at once determined to the extremities, and the ruptured vessel was thus closed.

A Botanic Guide to Health, A. I. Coffin, 1850

☞ Probably just pinching the nose did the trick, though the addition of pepper may have convinced the patient that he was taking some efficacious medicine. However, three quarts of blood is a lot to lose in one session; Dr Coffin (a widely trusted writer on medicine despite his name) does not say how long the patient took to recover after losing 60 per cent of his blood.

For a canker in the nose

Take old ale, and having boiled it on the fire, and cleansed it, add thereto a pretty quantity of live honey and as much alum, and then with a syringe or such like wash the sores therewith very warm.

The English Housewives' Household Physic, Gevase Markham, 1638

☞ Alum, being astringent and styptic, would have helped heal a canker (an open sore).

For rheum in the throat

Make a cap of brown paper, perfume it with frankincense, and apply it hot to the head, then take hard eggs, and lay them hot to the nape of the neck, and anoint the throat with oils of rice and sweet almonds, and lay your self to sweat; and after sweating mix syrup of roses, syrup of mulberries, and plantain water together, and gargle the throat therewith. In want of the said syrup use woodbine water.

The Queens Closet Opened, W.M., 1696

☞ Here is an example of treatment using brown paper, as specified in the nursery rhyme 'Jack and Jill'. It was more important that the paper was absorbent than brown. 'Rheum' was a watery mucus.

Canterbury bells (campanula)

The fresh tops, with the buds of the flowers upon them, contain most virtue, but the dried leaves may be used. An infusion of them sharpened with a few drops of spirit of vitriol, and sweetened with honey, is an excellent medicine for sore throats, used by way of a gargle. The plant is so famous for this virtue, that one of its common English names is throatwort; if the medicine be swallowed there is no great harm in it; but, in the use of every thing in this way, it is best to spit the liquor out together with the foulnesses which it may have washed from the affected parts.

The Useful Family Herbal, John Hill, 1754

☛ Canterbury bells (campanula), introduced into Britain in the sixteenth century, was one of a number of plants called 'throatwort' on account of their use for treating sore throats.

A bronchocele

Burnt sponge is a remedy for the bronchocele, in which cases it has been administered with success in the following manner. The stomach and bowels having been duly cleansed by a vomit and purge taken two days before, the patient, on going to bed, is to place a bolus, consisting of half a drachm of burnt sponge, and as much honey as is necessary, in the mouth, under the tongue, and as it gradually dissolves, to swallow it. This bolus is to be repeated for six succeeding nights. A bitter powder, made of five grains of chamomile flowers, gentian root, and the lesser centaury tops, is to be taken every seventh day during the use of the bolus, and on the eighth day the purge is to be repeated. Others have employed sponge, in these cases, in the form of a lozenge, which is certainly more conveniently held in the mouth than a bolus.

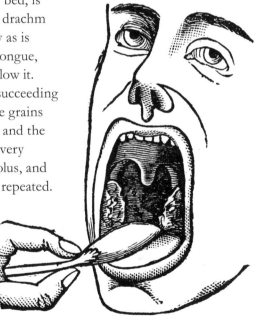

Thesaurus Medicaminum,
Richard Pearson, 1810

🖙 A 'bronchocele' is a swelling of the thyroid gland. This remedy has a long history – and sea-sponges do contain the necessary iodine to counter the deficiency which produces a goitre.

The thickening eclegma

Take oil of sweet almonds, one ounce; syrups of red poppy, of purslain, and of jujubes, and [the licking medicine called] *Lohor Sanum*, of each half an ounce; sugar-candy, a sufficient quantity. Mix them in a marble mortar for the space of an hour; and make a perfectly mixed licking medicine, which is to be kept in a galley-pot for use. It is to be taken frequently licking it off of a liquorice stick.

The Compleat Method of Curing Almost All Diseases, Thomas Sydenham, 1694

🖙 An 'eclegma' (or eclegme), was a linctus, a medicine to be licked or sucked, while a jujube was the fruit of a plant of the Zizyphus family.

First aid

THERE is evidence of healing after trepanation and bone-setting in prehistoric times, to show that first aid has a long history of success. But how many of us are still unsure how to stop a nosebleed, or whether you should suck the poison out of a snakebite?

To make oil of eggs

Take twelve yolks of eggs, and put them in a pot over the fire, and let them stand till you perceive them to grow black, then put them in a press and press out the oil. This oil is good for all manner of burning and scaldings whatever.

The Queens Closet Opened, W.M., 1696

🗫 Oil derived from the yolk of eggs is indeed very good for burns.

For him that hath a bunch on his head, or that hath his head swollen with a fall

Take an ounce of bay-salt, raw honey three ounces, cumin three ounces, turpentine two ounces; intermingle all this well upon the fire, then lay it upon a linnen cloth, and make thereof plasters, the which you shall lay hot to his head, and it will altogether assuage the swelling, and heal him clean and neat.

The Treasury of Hidden Secrets, 1659

🗫 A 'bunch' was a swelling or tumour. Cumin is effective against the inflammation caused by the crystallisation of uric acid in gout.

If apparently dead from noxious vapours, lightning, etc.

1. Remove the body into a cool fresh air.
2. Dash cold water on the face, neck, and breast frequently.
3. If the body be cold, apply warmth, as recommended for the apparently drowned.
4. In order to restore breathing, introduce the pipe of a common bellows into one nostril, carefully closing the other and mouth; at the same time drawing downwards, and pushing gently backwards, the upper part of the windpipe, to allow a free admission of air; blow the bellows gently, in order to inflate the lungs, till the breast be a little raised; the mouth and nostrils should then be set free, and a moderate pressure made with the hand upon the breast. Repeat this process till life appears.
5. Let Electricity (particularly in accidents from lightning) be early employed by a Medical Assistant.

The New Family Herbal, Matthew Robinson, 1869

🖙 The Royal Humane Society was founded in 1774 to promote the use of first aid and resuscitation, and mouth-to-mouth ventilation had been in use in Holland since the previous decade. It is curious to see the bellows, rather than mouth-to-mouth ventilation, recommended here 'where the apparatus of the [Royal Humane] Society is not at hand'.

An extended navel

A man had his navel standing out like to a man's yard; was healed with a thread dipped in the oil of vitriol, by tying the thread hard about it every day.

A Treatise of Chirurgery, Leonardo Fioravanti, 1652

🖙 A remedy taken from Paracelsus, the influential sixteenth-century Swiss physician. This appears to have been an inconveniently outward navel, possibly with some inflammation. The tightening thread alone would probably have done the trick, without the oil of vitriol, which is sulphuric acid.

Black plaster

Take of colophonia rosin, ship-pitch [tar], white wax, Roman vitriol, ceruss, olibanum, myrrh, of each eight ounces; oil of juniper berries three ounces; oil of roses seven ounces; oil of eggs two ounces; oil of spike [lavender] one ounce; white vitriol, red coral, mummy, of each two ounces; earth of Lemnos, mastic, dragons blood, of each an ounce; the fat of an heron, one ounce; the fat of timullus [a kind of fish], three ounces; lodestone prepared, two ounces; earthworms prepared, camphor, of each one ounce; make them into a plaster, according to art.

It is very good (say they) in green [fresh] wounds and pricks.

A Physical Directory, Nicholas Culpeper, 1651

☞ 'Dragons blood' was the resin from a palm, *Calamus draco*, which was imported from South America and the East Indies; 'lodestone' was magnetic iron oxide; 'Roman vitriol' was copper sulphate. None of these would have done much good. Culpeper's translation of the Royal College of Physicians' *Pharmacopoeia* is sprinkled with critical comments; his 'say they' may imply doubts in this remedy's power.

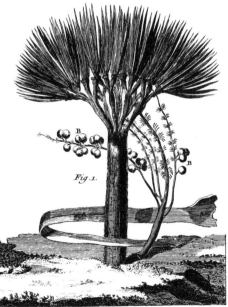

Fig. 1.

For one that is burned with gunpowder or otherwise

Take one handfull of groundsel, twelve heads of houseleek, one pint of
goose dung, as much chickens' dung, of the newest that can be gotten,
stamp the herbs as small as you can, then put the dung into a mortar,
temper them together with a pottle [pot] of boars' grease, labour them
together half an hour, and strain it through a canvas bag with a cleft
stick into an earthenware pan, and use it when need requireth; it will
last two year.

*A Choice Manual of Rare and Select Secrets in Physick
and Chyrurgery*, Elizabeth Grey, 1653

☞ It is curious that the recipe specifies the newest chicken dung but then
suggests that the mixture will keep adequately for two years, particularly
as no heat is being applied. Groundsel has been used since classical times
as a skin salve.

A lost nail

If a nail has come off a hand take wheaten grains, pound, mix with
honey place on the finger; boil black-thorn bark; wash with the liquid.

The Lacnunga, eleventh century

☞ The power of blackthorn to draw together soft tissues is well attested,
and together with the emollient of the wheat starch and the antibacterial
quality of honey this would have made a fairly effective treatment. Black-
thorn was believed to be particularly powerful because of its identification
as the material of Jesus' crown of thorns.

For an uncomb or sore finger

Shred one handful of smallage very small, and put to it one spoonful
of honey, the yolk of an egg, add a little wheat flower to make it thick;
then spread it on a cloth, and lay it to the sore twice a day.

The Queens Closet Opened, W.M., 1696

🌿 'Smallage' was angelica (wild celery) or water parsley, an infusion of which was used to wash and heal ulcers; with the protein of the egg and the antibacterial and antiseptic qualities of honey, this could have been quite helpful. Also known as an 'income', 'uncome' or 'ancome', an 'uncomb' was probably originally something that 'came on'; a visitation.

Bleeding of a wound

Take ripe puff-balls. Break them warily and save the powder. Strew this on the wound and bind it on. This will absolutely stop the bleeding of an amputated limb without any cautery.

Primitive Physick, John Wesley, 1755

🌿 Puffballs do indeed work as a styptic, and are recognized as having painkilling properties; but not many now would trust them to stop blood flow following an amputation.

For the bite of an adder

If adder or snake [venom] be within man or woman: stamp rue and urine and give [it to] the sick to drink. Or temper urine of the sick man or beast and arnement and make it some deal hard and give him [it] to drink and he shall cast him [vomit] with all the venom.

Rosa Medicinae, John of Gaddesden, fourteenth century

🌿 'Arnement' was ink or its constituents – mainly resin and soot. The idea of drinking urine as a medicine is historically widespread, though little used now in Europe. This is a curious recipe: crushed rue was used to relieve acid-based wasp stings, but the active constituent of adder venom is protein rather than acid. There may have been a perceived association between wasp sting and adder venom.

Grey ground liverwort (*Lichen cinereus terrestris*)

A plant very common by our dry wood-sides, and in pastures, in some degree resembling green liverwort, but differing in colour, and in its fructification.

The whole plant is used, and it has been of late very famous. Its efficacy is against the bite of a mad dog; it is mixed with pepper, and the person is at the same time to bathe in the sea. There have been instances of its success, when given to dogs, but perhaps no cure was ever performed upon a human creature when this terrible disease had arisen to any height. Bleeding and opium are the present practice.

The Useful Family Herbal, John Hill, 1754

🐾 Until Pasteur successfully tested a vaccine in 1885, rabies confounded all forms of treatment. As Hill points out, this treatment worked for dogs, but he doubts whether any treatment has worked for a human at the critical point of the disease.

To staunch the bleeding of a wound

Take a hound's turd, and lay that on a hot coal, and bind it [to the wound], and that shall staunch bleeding; or else bruise a long worm, and make powder of it, and cast it on the wound; or take the ear of a hare, and make powder thereof, and cast that on the wound, and that will staunch bleeding.

A Choice Manual of Rare and Select Secrets in Physick and Chyrurgery, Elizabeth Grey, 1653

🐾 This is a remedy with connotations of magic rather than medicine. Earthworms may have antibacterial properties, but burnt dog turds and powdered hares' ears are probably not a good idea.

A black eye

Convallaria (Solomon's Seal) – the juice from the fresh root will take away a 'black eye'.

Merck's Manual of the Materia Medica, 1899

☙ Long used as a treatment for bruises, *Convallaria racemosa* was the subject of this, one hopes, caustic comment in *Gerard's Herbal* of 1636: 'The roots of Solomon's Seal, stamped while it is fresh and green and applied, taketh away in one night or two at the most, any bruise, black or blue spots gotten by falls or women's wilfullness in stumbling upon their hasty husband's fists, or such like.'

To draw up the uvula

Take a new-laid egg, and roast it till it be blue, and then crush it between a cloth, and lay it to the crown of the head, and once in 12 hours lay new [repeat], till it be drawn up.

The Queens Closet Opened, W.M., 1696

☙ Deviation of the uvula to the right or left may be due to a stroke or an abscess in one tonsil. 'Drawing up' the uvula may have been an attempt to make it hang straight, though it is doubtful that the treatment described would have helped much.

Loose-strife or willow herb

This herb is good to stay all manner of bleeding at mouth or nose or wounds and all fluxes of the belly, and the bloody flux, given either to drink, or taken by clyster; it stayeth also the abundance of women's courses; it is a singular good wound herb for all green [fresh] wounds, to stay the bleeding, and quickly to close together the lips of the wound, if the herbs be bruised and the juice be quickly applied; it is often used in gargles for sore mouths, as also for the secret parts.

The English Physitian, Nicholas Culpeper, 1652

☙ Loosestrife, or willowherb, is indeed effective against diarrhoea, and as a gargle, and as a styptic for cuts.

To draw an arrow head, or other iron out of a wound

Take the juice of valerian, in the which you shall wet a tent [soft cloth], and put it into the wound, and lay the same herb stamped upon it, then your band or binding as appertaineth, and by this means you shall draw out the iron, and after heal the wound as it requireth.

A Choice Manual, Countess of Kent, 1708

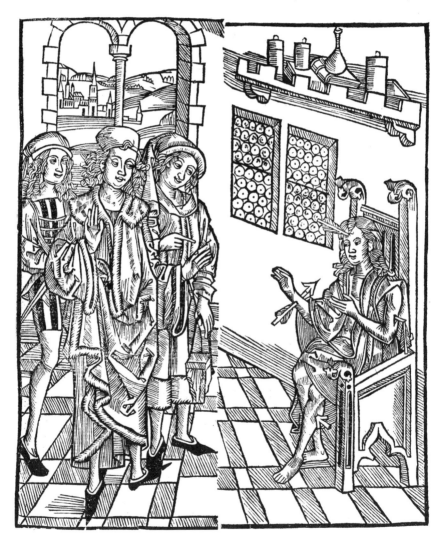

As a major non-prescription sedative, taken internally, valerian acts as a calmative on the nervous system; as a poultice, as described here, its power would be mostly antibacterial. An equivalent modern poultice for splinters is magnesium sulphate, though this would have trouble making anything as large as an iron arrowhead fall out.

For a wound

If there is iron or wood or thorn in any place of a man's body, take agrimony and stamp it with cold grease and lay it thereto, or take dittany and lay it thereto or drink it.

Rosa Medicinae, John of Gaddesden, fourteenth century

John of Gaddesden was the personal physician of Edward II, and is credited with curing the king's son of smallpox. He is thought to have been the model for the Doctor of Physick in Chaucer's *Canterbury Tales*. Agrimony has a long history as a treatment for flesh wounds, particularly on the battlefield.

For snakebite

TINCTURE OF VIRGINIA SNAKEROOT   Virginia snakeroot, well bruised, salt of tartar, beat all into a small powder in a hot iron mortar, and put into a glass matrass, and affuse [pour] thereon the best tartarised spirit of wine. Cover it with a blind head, luting the juncture, and digest for a month in a very gentle heat, shaking the glass once a day; then being fine decant the clear tincture for use.

It is one of the greatest antidotes and alexipharmacs [antidotes for poison] in the world, performing that which no other alexipharmac will do. It infallibly cures the biting of the rattle-snake (the most venomous of all serpents) and immediately secures the patient from death; its sanitive virtue being as volatile and swift as the volatility of and acuteness of the poison is fierce and dangerous.

Bates' Dispensatory, translated and edited by William Salmon (1694)

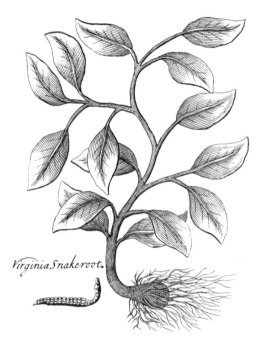

Virginia Snakeroot.

☞ 'Luting' the joint of the matrass (the flask) meant sealing it against the air – a 'blind head' was a secure cover. 'Digesting' here meant maturing through heat.

Snakeroot (there are many varieties found in North America) was an exciting discovery at the end of the seventeenth century, which promised to provide an instant cure for snakebites; Salmon draws attention to the similarity between the attributes of the poison and the antidote, a manifestation of the like-for-like concept that runs through the history of medicine from the doctrine of signatures to homoeopathy. Sadly there seems to be no scientific basis for the claims of snakeroot.

A direct approach to snake bites

The *National Intelligencer* a year or two since published a recipe for the cure of a rattlesnake bite, which it claimed was infallible … a daughter of Wm Reed of the town of Pittsfield, who was bitten on the arm some three years ago, was cured by drinking whisky until drunkenness and stupor were produced, and she has never felt any inconvenience from the bite since, which goes to show that whisky is sometimes useful.

The Book You Want: How to Cure Everything,
How to Do Everything, Receipts for Everything, John King 1885

☞ No side effects are here reported; more information would have been useful, for example the age of the female, and whether she was at all accustomed to whisky in the absence of rattlesnakes.

Contusions

Treatment. Bathe the part with vinegar lin. Sapon. Lin. Vol. Spt. mindereri, or arquebusade; and if necessary, apply a poultice of oatmeal and vinegar. If there be inflammation, bleed, and purge, use emollient fomentations and cataplasms. If suppuration appears, apply proper topical remedies to forward it, and treat as in abscesses.

The Medical Pocket Book, Boston, 1712

☞ This remedy was clearly to be administered only by a trained physician who would be able to understand the abbreviations, and the text shows how the use of pharmaceutical terms acknowledged the status of the professional. Such use of language was aped and parodied by quacks, such as the one noted by Ned Ward in *London Spy* (1698–1703), who refers to his authority as 'Doctor Honorificicabilitudinitatibusque', whose maxim is the meaningless 'Manus Sanaque in Cobile Sanaquorum'.

An 'arquebusade' was an ointment designed for the treatment of gunshot wounds; that part of the recipe is effectively offering the option 'put the appropriate ointment on it.'

A wonderful experience for the headache

Set a dish or platter of tin upon the bare head filled with water, put an ounce and a half or two ounces of molten lead therein while he hath it upon the head. Or else make a garland of vervain and wear it day and night; that helpeth wonderfully.

A Most Excellent and Perfect Homish Apothecarye, John Hollybush's translation of Hieronymus Braunschweig, 1561

☞ There cannot have been many, if any, who went for the first option. As a poultice vervain (verbena) is effective against headaches; it colours the skin red, so it was believed that the poultice therapeutically drew the blood away from the centre of the body.

GRIPING IN THE GUTS

POOR FOOD HYGIENE and unregulated cooking temperatures would have led to frequent gastric upheavals and what John Hollybush called 'outrageous sieges' (trips to/long sessions on the toilet); the occasional mention of 'running water' or 'fair water' in recipes indicates an awareness of the danger of disease from standing or unclean water.

Of flatulence, or wind

All nervous patients, without exception, are afflicted with wind or flatulencies in the stomach or bowels, which arises chiefly from the want of tone or vigour in these organs. Crude flatulent aliment, such as dried flesh, beans, coleworts, cabbages, and such like, may increase this complaint; but strong and healthy people are seldom troubled with wind, unless they either overload their stomachs, or drink liquors that are in a fermenting state, and consequently full of elastic air. While therefore the matter of flatulence proceeds from our aliments, the cause which makes air separate from them in such quantity as to occasion complaints is almost always a fault of the bowels themselves, which are too weak to prevent the production of elastic air, or to expel it after it is produced.

For strengthening the stomach and bowels, and consequently for lessening the production of flatulence, Doctor Whytt recommends the Peruvian bark, bitters, chalybeates, and exercise. In flatulent cases he thinks some nutmeg or ginger should be added to the tincture of bark and bitters, and that the aromatic powder should be joined with the filings of iron.

Domestic Medicine, William Buchan, 1774

☞ Buchan's assured tone must have been of some comfort to his readers; perhaps the desire for the development of tone and vigour in the stomach and bowels did indeed lead some of them to abandon drinks that were full of elastic air.

For a lask

Take the nether jaw of a pike, seeth it to a powder and drink it.

A Choice Manual of Rare and Select Secrets in Physick and Chyrurgery, Elizabeth Grey, 1653

☞ 'Lask' was diarrhoea. Curiously, this is not the only recipe from around this time which uses the jaw of a pike. In 1671 John Archer, physician to the king, recommended the meat of the pike for invalids, it being 'easily distributed' (around the body).

The streight gut

Is often infested with little white flat worms, call'd Ascarides, which are destroyed by the following clyster: boil quicksilver in water in an earthenware pot for two hours; give by way of clyster.

The Ancient Physician's Legacy to his Country, Thomas Dover, 1733

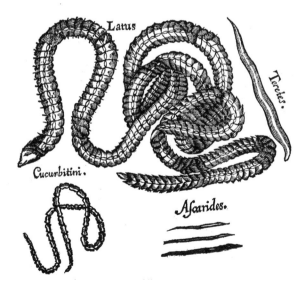

☞ Ascarides are parasitic roundworms that infest the gut, causing obstruction and sometimes even completely blocking the alimentary canal. Modern medicines for getting rid of them still contain mercury (quicksilver).

To cure a great flux or looseness in the belly

Take a hard egg and peel off the shell, and put the smaller end of it hot to the fundament or arsehole, and when that is cold take another such hot, fresh, hard, and peeled egg, and apply it as aforesaid.

The Queens Closet Opened, W.M., 1696

☞ A remedy that might have given some comfort, though it is hard to see how it would have cured diarrhoea.

For diarrhoea

Against diarrhoea: take a hen's egg; lay it in vinegar for two nights; if it does not split, tap it a little; put it back in the vinegar for one night; beat it then in butter; put it in oil; then put a little above the fire; give it to eat.

The Lacnunga, eleventh century

☞ This seems to be basically a recipe for a small omelette, recognized as sensible food for someone suffering from diarrhoea.

Electuary lenitive (for the poor)

Polypodie of the oak, bruised, 3 oz, fennel seeds ½ oz, betony, agrimony, adianthos, politric, scolopendry, of each 2 handfuls, leaves of senna, cleansed, 2 oz, aniseeds, ½ oz, pulp of cassia, pulp of tamarinds, and of prunes, of each 6 oz; senna in powder with aniseeds 4½ oz; a pound of sugar.

For the poor it should have senna cleansed, 2 oz, aniseeds ½ oz, pulp of prunes and tamarinds 9 oz each, senna in powder with aniseeds 4½ oz, sugar 1 lb.

The Charitable Physician, Philbert Guibert, 1639

An 'electuary' was a medicinal paste, while a 'lenitive' was a mild laxative. Guibert's approach of supplying two remedies, one for the rich and one for the poor, is commendable, but readers should take into account that a building labourer's daily wage in 1639 was less than the cost of a pound of sugar. The 'polypodie of oak' was a fern found growing on oak trees, while 'scolopendry' was the hart's-tongue fern.

A remedy for colic

Earwax is accounted a most present remedy for the colic (if taken in drink).

The History of Animals as They are Useful in Physick and Chirurgery, John Schroder, 1659

Human body parts and products were taken more commonly in early-modern medicine than is often thought. Schroder's book discusses them on a par with those from animals.

Rhubarb

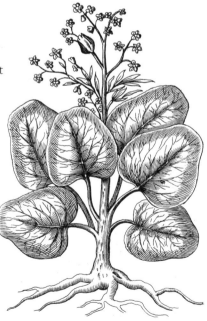

The root is good against the windiness, wambling, and weakness of the stomach, and all pain thereof, and it is good against cramps, the griefs of the liver and milt, gnawing and griping of the belly, kidneys, and bladder, the ache of the breasts and mother, the sciatica, spitting of blood, sobbing, hicket, the bloody-flux and lask, the fits of fevers, all stingings and venomous bitings; one dram, taken in a fever with hydromel for the same purposes; and with Syrupus Acetosus [medicated syrup], against the griefs of the liver and milt.

The Garden of Health, William Langham, 1578

🐦 The 'milt' was the spleen, and remains a common word for the spleen of animals today, while 'wambling of the stomach' was an upset tummy. The 'mother' in this context was the uterus. Langham was fulsome in his praise for rhubarb: 'Life and health to preserve, use to eat rhubarb daily.'

A present medicine for the hickop

Take thy finger ends, and stop both thine ears very hard, and the hickop will surcease immediately.

A Rich Storehouse, or Treasurie for the Diseased, 1607

🐦 I tried it, and it worked.

Of yelking or hicket

Yelking is a motion of the stomach, and it is as it were a cramp of the stomach raised of the expulsive virtue, which goeth about to thrust forth evil and hurtful things. This disease is caused for the most part, either of fulness or of emptiness, as Hippocrates witnesseth ... Also coldness of the mouth of the stomach, and corruption of the food causeth yelking, which causeth children to have the hicket often.

When yelking is engendered of coldness, you must lay upon the stomach wool dipped in the oil wherein hath been sodden rue, cumin, and wormwood. Also oil of mastic, and of *Castoreum* being anointed doth profit. To children warm linen cloths being applied too do help often. They that be of full age, minister to them wine to drink, or apum sodden in *Aqua mulsa*, or cumin beaten, or asarum, or pennyroyal, each of these by himself, or else mixed with other. Moreover, holding of the breath which doth increase heat, is a present remedy for them that do yelk through cold.

The Method of Physick, Philip Barrough, 1639

🐦 'Yelking' and 'hicket' (as well as 'yexing') were hiccoughs or hiccups – and much better words to describe this affliction. 'Apum' here may be 'apium', a genus of plants including celery and marshwort; 'aqua mulsa' was honey dissolved in water. These remedies may have been for chronic hiccupping; it was presumably not thought necessary to simply recommend a glass of water.

The Lady Drury's medicine for the colic, proved

Take a turf of green grass, and lay it to the navel, and let it lie till you find ease; the green side must be laid next to the belly.

The Queens Closet Opened, W.M., 1696

☞ A pleasant – if perhaps inconvenient – way of cooling the lower abdomen.

A laxative tisane, with senna, rhubarb, and agaric

Take ¾ of a pint of good water in the which boil and scum ... an ounce of liquorice, then take it from the fire and infuse in it all night a little bag with half an ounce of senna and aniseeds, in the which enclose also the weight of a dram and a half of rhubarb with a little cinnamon, and as much agaric with a little ginger bruised; the morning following strain and press it through a linen cloth, and this shall be suitable for twice taking.

The Charitable Physician, Philbert Guibert, 1639

☞ The 'agaric' here is probably white agaric, *Polyporus officinalis*, long used in medicine as an irritant to the stomach and intestines, but primarily as a suppressor of sweating. Combined with the calming effect of ginger on the gut, the agaric would have provided a mild laxative effect.

An excellent extract of Mars, for diarrhœas and fluxes

Take filings of steel (which you may buy at the needle-makers), put them in a well-glazed pipkin, and pour thereon a quart of good deep-red wine (that which is used to colour white-wine), let it boil until about three parts of the wine be consumed, stirring often with an iron spatula. Then strain it while it is hot.

It is a great and certain remedy for dysenteries, diarrhœas, old hepatical fluxes, and such like diseases; you may give an ounce of it in broth fasting, for some mornings together. This I have sufficiently experienced with happy success.

A Choice Collection of Rare Secrets and Experiments,
collected by Sir Kenelm Digby, 1682

☞ The broth alone, given while fasting, might have been a more helpful treatment for diarrhoea. Another way of taking iron was through drinking 'smiths forge-water', the water blacksmiths used for cooling red-hot iron. Iron was long thought to be good for loose bowels, but modern iron supplements often carry warnings about diarrhoea as a side effect.

For the wind in the veins

Take powder of liquorice, caraway seed and sugarcandy beaten small, of each an equal quantity to your taste, to which put rhubarb in powder a third part or more, with as much cream of tartar pulverised; put it in a box, and keep it in your pocket, and eat as much of it as will lie on a sixpence, twice or thrice in a day for a week together; this will gently purge you, cool the blood, and expel the wind out of the veins. This hath helped those that have not been able to go.

The Queens Closet Opened, W.M., 1696

☞ Clearly this is to do with constipation, as indicated by the rhubarb and the euphemism at the end. But 'wind' could affect any part of the body – the heart or muscles as well as any part of the alimentary canal.

For indigestion

Take white chalk 2 drams, crabs-eyes 1 dram, nutmegs 1 dram, white sugar 12 drams, mucilage of quince-seeds the same. Mix and make tablets.

1) You may eat 1 or 2 drams or more at a time, as you eat sugar-plums, and they will (by reason they are made of a fixed alcali) absorb

the acid humor which is the cause of those intolerable gnawing pains at stomach.

2) This is made for such as cannot take the medicine without sugar; but to speak truth, the alcalies alone are much more effectual.

Bates' Dispensatory, translated and edited by William Salmon, 1694

☞ Salmon's description of stomachache is all too recognizable. 'Crabs' eyes' was at this time a term for the small concretions of carbonate of lime found in the stomachs of crustacea; they were used medically as an antacid.

Dyspepsia

Treatment – Take – no, just stop taking. "Throw all medicine to the dogs." Yes, and food also. What, starve? No, but simply get hungry; whoever heard of a dyspeptic being hungry? At least those who eat three meals a day. They eat because victuals taste good – mouth-hunger, only.

The Book You Want: How to Cure Everything,
How to Do Everything, Receipts for Everything, John King, 1885

☞ This advice is full of infectious enthusiasm and self-belief. But you might not be consulting a book with this title if you wanted a scientific approach.

A last resort

☞ When all else failed, suppositories have been available throughout history.

An onion put in as a suppository, purgeth the emerods [haemorrhoids], and draweth down the flowers.

The Garden of Health, William Langham, 1578

If thou be costive – If a man or woman be too fast bounden that none of these things may help them: take a pipe of elerne [common elder] as great as a spindle or some deal more and do it in his fundament an handbreadth deep.

Corpus Compendium, 1330

Take a beet root, or a cabbage root, cut it according to the length and shape of your fore-finger, that is, taper; only a little pointed at one end; dust it about with a little salt powdered fine, and put it up your fundament.

The Family-Physician and the House-Apothecary, Gideon Harvey, 1676

WATERWORKS

I T IS EASY to see why people were obsessed with bladder stones; diets with a regular intake of alcohol and the absence of clean water to flush out waste products from the system led to high incidence of gout, which can cause stones in the bladder. The most noticeable symptom of this was what William Langham called 'stopped pipes'. Any avenue was explored that might obviate the need for removal of the stones by surgery or forceps.

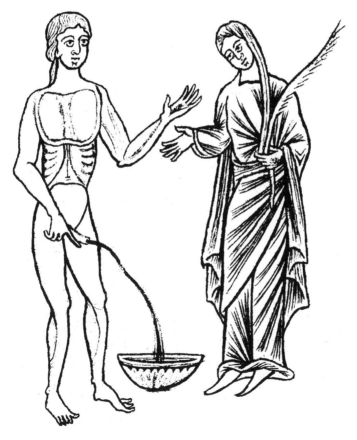

For the stopping of the urine

Take the shells of quick snails, wash them and dry them clean, and beat them into fine powder; whereof take a pretty quantity in white-wine or thin broth.

The Queens Closet Opened, W.M., 1696

☞ 'Quick' snails were live ones. Snail shells are composed almost entirely of calcium carbonate, itself a component of many human bladder stones, so this recipe is unlikely to have helped.

To make one piss

Take the powder of the berries of ivy, and drink it with white wine, or else with stale ale hot.

The Widdowes Treasure, 1639

☞ Ground ivy has long been known as a diuretic; usually the juice of the roots was used, though Galen had located the healing powers of the plant in its flowers.

Surgery for the stone

In Petty France, Westminster, at a house with a black door and a red knocker, between the sign of the Rose and Crown, is a German who hath a powder which with the blessing of God upon it certainly cures the stone; and for those that have decided to be cut for it, it wonderfully dissolves great stones in the kidneys and bladder, and brings them away by urine, with much ease and safety.

Handbill, *c.* 1700

☞ A clear indication that surgery was a common recourse, but also that patients had a choice of treatment that avoided surgery. Many quack doctors claimed to be German at this time.

SPORTING IN THE
GARDEN OF VENUS

H EALTH issues to do with sexual functions included impotence and contraception as well as venereal disease. Syphilis, seen either as just desserts for fornication, or unfair punishment for harmless fun, occupied the minds of moralists as well as physicians.

An incidental aphrodisiac

Radish sodden in wine and drunk morn and even, breaketh and expelleth the stone, openeth the gall, diminisheth the spleen, and moveth Venus.

The Garden of Health, William Langham, 1578

It is to be hoped that these effects were not simultaneous.

An exceedingly good ointment for the French pox

Take a quarter of a pint of hog's grease unfried, an ounce of quicksilver, and qualify the quicksilver with fasting spittle, and then put unto the hog's grease and quicksilver four or five spoonfuls of vinegar that is both strong and sharp, and then heat-temper them altogether, for the space of two or three hours together; and then put it into some earthenware pot or gallipot and so keep it close stopped, whereby neither dust nor any other thing may come to hurt it; and when occasion serveth for the use thereof, let the diseased person be anointed therewith very often before a good fire, and doubtless he shall find great ease thereby in a short space.

A Rich Storehouse, or Treasurie for the Diseased, 1607

By Doctor _James Tilborgh_, Famous through _Germany_, and _Holland_, _Brabant_, _France_ and _Italy_, for Curing the FRENCH POX, and all _Venereal Distempers_; Living at present at the _Black-Swan_ in St. _Giles's_ in the Fields, over against _Drury-Lane_ End, where you shall see at Night three Lanthorns with Candles burning in them upon the Belcony: Where he may be spoke with all a-lone, from Eight of the Clock in the Morning, till Ten at Night, desiring you to be careful for your own benefit not to mistake the place because there is a new person that is lately come over and hath presumed to make use of the Bill and Peice which formerly I did make use of. And further without any name, which is the cause I have altered my Peice. And I desire nothing for my labour and pain till the person be cured, and wish you to be careful and not be abused.

THis is to give notice by these Papers, That there is a very expert famous outlandish Doctor, and Citizen of _Hambourgh_, who is lately arrived here in _London_, and hath brought by Gods blessing, a wonderful Art with him, which he hath found through long seeking for, and travelling through many Kingdoms, yet not without great trouble and charge. _viz._ The right way of Curing the Pox, otherwise called _Morbum Gallicum_, with all its dependants, which no man can so soundly Cure as he; which he hath shewn to many thousands. And because it is the best time of the year to Cure such Diseases, he hath caused these Bills to be Printed

FIRST, He Cures the _French Pox_, with all its dependents, _viz_. The Running of the Reins, Pains in the Groin, and in making of water, Shankers, Buboes, Scabdkloat, Spanish Kraagen, Boils and Scabbs about the Head, Holes in the Throat and Neck, and rotting of the Palate and Grisdels of the Nose and Gums, whereby the Nose and the Palate often times comes to fall, and by that means Men are bereaved of their speech all their

☞ French pox was syphilis, for which mercury (quicksilver) was the standard treatment. In this recipe it is qualified (diluted) with the saliva of someone who is fasting.

French pox

THE CORALLINE SECRET   It is made of crude mercury, spirit of nitre distilled therefrom with cohobations [redistillation], so will the arcanum [elixir] remain in the bottom, which is to be edulcorated [softened] either by calcinations or washing it with water.

If the reducing of the mercury into small particles accidentally add to the virtue of the mercury, by enlarging the surface thereof, if then by adding three times the quantity of spirit the particles be made three times as small, it follows by parity of reason, that its virtues must be three times as great.

Bates' Dispensatory, translated and edited by William Salmon, 1694

☞ Salmon's explanation seems to be taking the process away from alchemy and towards science, by observation and reason; but the assessment which follows – 'It brings forth all noxious humours in French Pox, leprosy, King's Evil, etc' – shows the persistence of the Galenic system. 'Calcination' meant reducing something to a powder by extreme heat.

A cure for the clap

For the full satisfaction of all those who have been sporting in the garden of Venus, and in seeking for pleasure have met with a clap or gonorrhea, I do promise to cure them in 8 or 9 days time … Also the cancer, or Noli me Tangere in the breast, or any other part of the body.

Handbill, Cornelius Tilbury, *c.* 1700

☞ 'Noli me tangere' was the name given to skin eruptions which often spread from basal cell carcinomas, with the term being in use from medieval times. The phrase was taken from the Vulgate (the Latin version of the Bible), from the scene where Jesus tells Mary Magdalen not to touch him; other names used were 'Jacob's ulcer' and 'rodent ulcer'.

A contraceptive for a gentleman

Hemp seed consumeth and dryeth so much that if it be eaten in great quantity, it dryeth seed of generation; it is hard to be digested, and maketh the head ache.

Approved Medicines and Cordiall Receiptes, Thomas Newton, 1580

☞ Within the Galenic system of humours hemp was seen as having drying powers. Clearly in the sixteenth century *Cannabis sativa* had pronounced effects, as *Cannabis indica* still does.

Of the loss of carnal copulation

They which be married, and cannot use the act of generation because of the sluggish impotency and weakness of their members, coming of a cold distemper wherewith they be vexed, or of some other cause, such ought to exercise the nether parts, and to use meats that do heat, and engender good humours; such as, the flesh of hens, capons, partridge, pheasants, young doves, birds of mountains, and specially sparrows, cock stones, and such like. Not only good nourishing meats, but windy meats are good for him, as be chickpeas, peas, beans, scallions, leeks, the root and seed of parsnips, pine nuts, sweet almonds, rape roots, and such other like. Also the eggs of partridges do stir up carnal lust. Let the patient sleep in a soft bed, and let him read things that do stir up lust, or let him hear them read. Let his privy members be continually chafed and rubbed with oils, ointments and other heating medicines.

Among simple medicines, these that follow do chiefly stir up carnal lust, as be rocket, mustard seed, garden cresses, nettle seed, root of aron, and pepper, *Satyrion, Orminum,* aniseed, squill, *Orchu,* called also *Testiculum canis,* whose greatest round root drunk with milk doth provoke stiffness of the yard. The stones of a fox dried, beaten to powder and drunk, do cause a stiffness of the member, not hurtful nor vain.

The Method of Physick, Philip Barrough, 1639

☙ The 'stones' of a fox, and earlier a cock, in this text are the testicles. 'Squill' is a sea onion, while 'aron' is an earlier version of arum; 'orminum' was the wild clary, and 'satyrion' and 'orchu' were kinds of orchid. This is clearly an application of the doctrine of signatures, given the shape of the onion or orchid tuber and stalk; in fact 'orchid' derives from the Greek word for a testicle.

A cure for impotence

A certain man called Bartholomew, having carnal company with his wife, could void no sperm at his yard, but only wind, the which by often using oleum vitrioli [oil of vitriol], with the spirit of tartar in distilled wine, and afterward the extraction of satirion, he performed the act very well.

A Treatise of Chirurgery, Leonardo Fioravanti, 1652

☙ 'Extraction of satirion' came from an orchid (see above), while 'spirit of tartar' was obtained by dry-distilling the crust from the sides of wine casks. Presumably this mixture was rubbed on, rather than drunk.

Mother and child

WHILE most licensed medical practice was in the hands of men, many conditions specific to women were treated by women. In around 1700 in London, Anne Davenport advertised her skill in treating 'any distemper incident to woman-kind'. Her address was given, unfortunately perhaps, as by 'the Coffin and Child, against the Watch House, Southampton Square'.

For a woman that hath her flowers too much

Take a hare's foot, and burn it, make powder of it, and let her drink it with stale ale.

A Choice Manual of Rare and Select Secrets in Physick and Chyrurgery, Elizabeth Grey, 1653

🐾 Hares' feet turn up occasionally in this book, and were (and are) used as amulets; in March 1665 Samuel Pepys attributed his resistance to cramp to carrying a hare's foot.

For the rising of the mother

Take columbine-seed and parsnip-seed of each three spoonfuls; beat them to fine powder, and boil them in a quart of ale to a pint, seething it with one handful of sage cut small; strain it, and drink it off warm every morning and evening, especially when you feel pain. And take two ounces of galbanum, spread it upon a cloth, and lay it upon the woman's navel.

The Queens Closet Opened, W.M., 1696

🐾 A woman's navel was supposed to have a direct connection to the 'mother' (uterus); early theories of anatomy proposed a system of veins

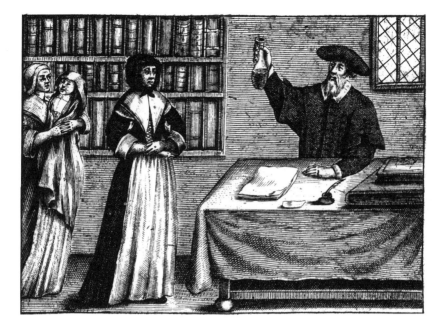

running the length of the body, with two connecting the navel and the genitals. Thus many gynaecological treatments of this period involve laying something on this area.

Barren-wort epidemium

It was an opinion with the old writers, that this plant produced no flowers; but the occasion is easily known. When it stands exposed to sun, it seldom does flower; we see that in gardens where it is planted in such situations, for it will stand many years without flowering; but our woods favour it, being dark and damp; the old people saw it in warmer climates, and under an unfavourable exposure. They called it from this circumstance, as well as from its virtue, by a name, which expressed being barren and fruitless.

The people in the north give milk in which the roots have been boiled, to the females of the domestic animals when they are running after the males, and they say that it has the certain effect of stopping the natural emotions. Plain sense leads these sort of people to many things; they have from this been taught to give it to young women of robust health subject to violent hysteric complaints, and I am assured with great success; they give the decoction of the root made strong and sweetened. 'Twas a coarse allusion that led them to the practice. It is said that, if they take it in too large quantity, it renders them stupid, but no ill consequence has attended this.

The Useful Family Herbal, John Hill, 1754

🖝 The proposal is that as the plant often produces no flowers it must have a tendency towards barrenness; the doctrine of signatures leads people to use the plant to suppress opposite tendencies, i.e. licentiousness, in both animals and women. 'Stupid' at this time meant 'stupefied' rather than 'idiotic'. Hill's description of this herb's use betrays a male urge to suppress any untoward behaviour by women – the Greek word for 'womb', *hystera*, is the origin of the word 'hysteria', showing a connection between the organ and the idea of 'female emotion'.

To prevent miscarrying

Lay a toast, sopped [soaked] in muscadel to her navel, and many times it doth good for it is a good medicine. But to take a little garden tansy, and having bruised it, sprinkle it with muscadel, and apply that to the navel, for it is better.

A Directory for Midwives, Nicholas Culpeper, 1652

🖝 Tansy was much used in menstruation treatments. Note that Culpeper states the quantity to be used; when used externally tansy can be dangerous to the skin.

Breast cancer

A certain woman having a corroding ulcer in the left breast with great pains, by means that she had not her natural sickness, she had also in the right breast, neck, and armpit, certain kernels, and hard tumours; and chiefly the left arm was astonied [paralysed] and taken; to whom sundry times I gave a purgation of the extraction of rhubarb, and the oil of gold, by the space of a month; outwardly I washed the breast with the decoction of the roots of celandine in wine; also I laid thereon pleggets wet with *oleum veneris*, mixed with honey, and rolled it; and afterward I laid on it our common opodeldoc, and so she was perfectly cured.

A Treatise of Chirurgery, Leonardo Fioravanti, 1652

☞ A 'plegget' was a compress, while *oleum veneris* was a complex alchemical composition based on copper. An 'opodeldoc' was a word for a plaster, invented by Paracelsus, usually a liniment of soap dissolved in alcohol, with essence of wormwood. Celandine has long been used in Russia in treatments for cancer.

To increase milk

Parsnip roots and fennel roots sodden in broth of chickens and afterwards eaten with a little fresh butter maketh your milk increase. Crystal made in fine powder, and mixed with as much fennel seed and sugar; drink it warm with a little wine.

The Widdowes Treasure, 1639

☞ The first proposal sounds as pleasant as the second sounds dangerous; it is difficult to see how ground crystal might be thought to increase milk.

A powder to stop the menses at the turn of life

Take alum two drams, japan earth one dram, pound in a mortar to a fine powder, divide into eight doses, take two a day.

The Family Physician, Edward Bullman, 1789

☞ 'Japan earth' was catechu, assumed in the seventeenth century to be an 'earth' (mineral), but in fact obtained from the bark, wood or fruits of various trees; it is astringent, so possibly reduces blood flow.

All in the mind

Not all early treatments for mental illness involved cutting open the head, incarceration or barely disguised punishment. Several made use of relieving or comforting herbs and lifestyle changes.

Against weakness of the brain and coldness thereof

Seethe rosemary in wine and let the patient receive the smoke at his nose and keep his head warm.

The Great Herbal, 1526

🐛 'Smoke' here is the vapour produced by heating. The immediate effect would be ingestion of the alcohol.

Bearsfoot or black hellebore

Bearsfoot was esteemed by the Ancients good for melancholy and madness, to purge the black choler and humours arising thence.

A Curious Herbal, Elizabeth Blackwell, 1737

🐛 Black hellebore (bearsfoot) carries two strong poisons. Its narcotic effect is probably why it was used for nervous disorders, as a sedative.

Vertigo

Symptoms. Objects, though at rest, seem to turn round; dimness of sight; and fear of falling.

Treatment. Bleed in the jugular, and cup in the back part of the head; blisters kept open; a vomit, and laxatives; then the nervous medicines, and chalybeate waters.

A Medical Pocket Book, John Elliot, 1798

☛ The treatment seems to involve a major assault on the patient's head. 'Nervous' medicines are those directed at the nerves, while 'chalybeate' (iron-rich) waters were recommended for many conditions, including melancholy, hysteria and 'an over-moist brain'.

Against frenzy

The juice of smallage or vinegar or oil of violets or roses, put together in a glass over the fire, and hot lay it to the patient's head, but first shave it.

The Great Herbal, 1526

☛ Frenzy, used at first in the sense of 'delirium', developed the medical meaning of 'inflammation of the brain', which in turn came to be known as meningitis.

Of whirling in the head

Many [there] are whom the head whirleth so sore, that he thinketh the earth turneth upside down; the same also hath pain in the eye, he thinketh that a sort of flies do fly before his eyes; those may be healed of this wise; they may drink no strong drinks nor wine without it be well allayed with water, and so then ought to be given pills made of half an ounce of aloe, and a pennyweight of mastic; give him of them every night five, the bigness of small beans, and give him after the Diamargariton or dianthus or else diaphiris, for the same comfort the head and stomach; and anoint his head with oil of camomile.

A Most Excellent and Perfect Homish Apothecarye,
John Hollybush's translation of Hieronymus Braunschweig, 1561

☛ This seems to be a case of migraine; the recommendation to abstain from alcohol is wise. 'Diamargariton' was another name for 'manus Christi', a drink given to poorly people, consisting of rosewater or violet water mixed with sugar.

Of melancholy

This disease is a weakness of the mind, without being deprived of intellect, which renders people unhappy in the midst of pleasure, and often deprives them of performing the duties of life; the cause may be from the stoppage of any usual evacuation, from grief, intense study, narcotic or stupefactive poisons, the striking of eruptions, [such] as the scurvy, scrophula, or from too much solitude; or a fever on the spirits, obstruction of the menses, etc. The symptoms are a dread and horror of mind, with unusual depressing thoughts of things never likely to happen; a love of solitude, to indulging every crowding idea which succeeds each other and aggravates this disease …

Medicine – take honey, four ounces, rosemary finely powdered, an ounce, powder of valerian, four drams, powder of russia castor, one dram, musk in powder, twenty grains; mix well and take one teaspoonful twice a day; drink after a cup of featherfew tea.

The Family Physician, Edward Bullman, 1789

☞ 'Featherfew' is a very old corruption of the usual name 'feverfew'; the name indicates how the plant was used in medicine, to treat fevers. While this is a fairly astute assessment of what would now be called depression, it is notable that the first given possible source is constipation; should we think of this as an indication of what might reasonably be called the English 'disease', namely an obsession – which lasted well into the twentieth century – with emptying the bowels?

Lethargy

It is necessary for lethargics that people talk loudly in their presence. Tie their extremities lightly and rub their palms and soles hard; and let their feet be put in salt water up to the middle of their shins, and pull their hair and nose, and squeeze the toes and fingers tightly, and cause pigs to squeal in their ears … Put a feather, or a straw, in his nose to compel him to sneeze, and do not ever desist from hindering him from sleeping; and let human hair or other evil-smelling thing be

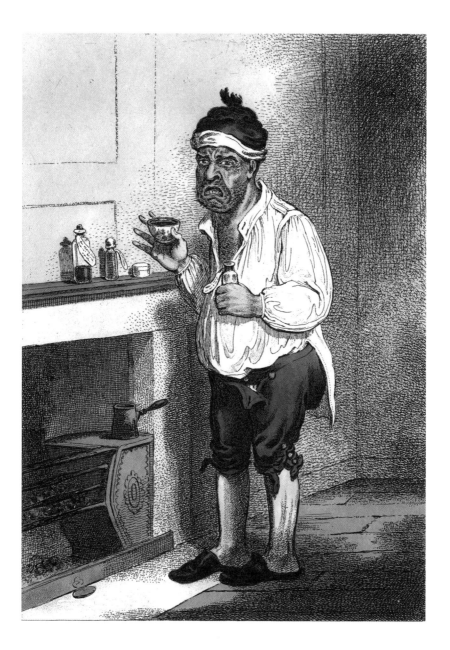

burnt under his nose. Apply, moreover, the cupping horn between the shoulders, and let a feather be put down his throat, to cause vomiting, and shave the back of the head, and rub oil of roses and vinegar and smallage [angelica] thereon.

Rosa Medicinae, John of Gaddesden, fourteenth century

🙾 The energy applied to the treatment has to be admired; only a very determined 'lethargic' would persist in the condition in the face of treatment of this order.

Of memory lost

Memoria deperdita, the loss of memory chanceth sometime alone, and sometime reason is hurt with it. It is caused of the lethargy and other soporiferous diseases. It cometh to pass also that the soporiferous diseases being ended, there ensueth forgetfullness.

As touching the cure, if loss of memory be caused by vehement purgations, or other immoderate evacuations, or by swounding [fainting] often, and so overmuch dryness do hurt the memory, then minister no medicine, but only restore the body by good diet. For the body being corroborate and strength renewed, the memory will come again.

The Method of Physick, Philip Barrough, 1639

🙾 'Corroborate' here means 'strengthened'. The idea of restoring memory by good diet might comfort many of the older generation; certainly the remedy would do little harm.

Of common madness

This disease proceedeth from a too vivid and exalted constitution of the blood. There is also another sort of madness that comes after long intermitting fevers and at length degenerates into folly, which is caused by the weakness and flatness of the blood, proceeding from a long fermentation thereof. You must therefore prescribe cordials, such as Treacle of Andromachus, the Electuary de Ovo, the Countesses Powder, Sir Walter Rawleigh's Powder in plague water, treacle water, or some other convenient vehicle. And enjoin a restorative diet.

In young persons let a vein be opened in the arm, and eight or nine ounces of blood taken away twice or thrice, every fourth day.

Then let the jugular veins be once opened. After which the whole cure depends upon the use of the following purging medicine, which must be given every third or fourth day while the disease lasts. But in the mean time it is to be observed that after the patient hath been purged eight or nine times, the exhibition of the electuary medicine must be omitted for a week or two.

Take of the domestic medicine (that is white bryony roots) in powder one dram, in cow's milk four ounces.

The Compleat Method of Curing Almost All Diseases,
Thomas Sydenham, 1694

☞ The extent of purging as a medical practice is indicated by the fact that a purging medicine is known as the 'domestic medicine'. The 'Countesses Powder' and 'Sir Walter Rawleigh's Powder' were formulas documented in recipe books made for the Countess of Kent and Sir Walter Raleigh. The 'Treacle of Andromachus' was the same as Venice treacle, a molasses-based poison-antidote, while the 'Electuary de Ovo' was the same but with baked egg yolk, herbs and spices.

To make a child merry

Hang a bundle of mugwort or make smoke thereof under the child's bed for it taketh away any annoyance for them.

The Great Herbal, 1526

☞ Infusions of mugwort (*Artemisia vulgaris*) were a traditional treatment for fits, as quoted by many writers; William Langham, the herbalist, fifty years later repeated the recommendation for the use of smoke. John Gerard, writing in 1597, noted the tendency among 'the Antient Writers' to ascribe to mugwort all-healing or 'fantastical' properties, which he dismissed as 'tending to witchcraft and sorcery, and to the great dishonour of God'.

Raging madness

Apply to the head clothes dipt in cold water;
Or, set the patient with his head under a great water-fall, as long as his strength will bear; or, pour water on his head out of a tea-kettle;
Or, let him eat nothing but apples for a month.

Primitive Physick, John Wesley, 1755

☞ Wesley's 'if that doesn't work, try this' approach, not entirely abandoned in current medical practice, is at least an attempt to try to treat insanity, at a time when many sufferers would simply be shut away from society. The range of water treatment, from gentle to violent, is confusing; apples are extremely good for the digestion and general wellbeing, though a month-long apple diet might drive anyone to distraction.

Hypochondriasis

Symptoms are generally low-spiritedness (the disorder being chiefly in the imagination), heaviness, oppression, and despondency; yet at times uncommon cheerfulness and flow of spirits; timidity, anxiety, fear, dread of dying, short cough, difficult breath, flatulency, pale urine, pains in the head, odd fancies, spasms.

Treatment. Bark and other tonics, nervous antispasmodics, such as castor, valerian, asa foetida, etc; attenuants, such as volatile salts and spirits; bitters and chalybeates if no fever; emetics, aperients, opiates, issues, and blisters, discretionally; the cold bath and chalybeate waters, food light and easy of digestion, cheerful company, and gentle exercise.

A Medical Pocket Book, John Elliot, 1798

☞ The last elements of the treatment sound the most sensible; 'issues' were blood-lettings, while 'aperients' were laxatives. Hypochondriasis in the eighteenth century was generally believed to derive from a digestive disorder, hence the use of castor and aperients, as well as the sedative valerian and the antispasmodic 'asa foetida'.

A heaviness of spirits

If you feel a heaviness or oppression of spirits, a quick pulse and shortness of breath, open a vein for ventilation, and you will find alleviation and refreshment.

A Treasury of Choice Medicines External and Internal, Julius Degravere, 1662

☞ This sounds like a self-treatment, administered with the casual air of reaching for an aspirin, which gives some idea of the widespread use of blood-letting.

Lettuce for sweet dreams

A common plant in our kitchen gardens, which we use to eat raw.

The juice of lettuce, is a good medicine to procure sleep, or the thick stalk eaten will serve the same purpose. It is a good method [for those] who require a gentle opiate, and will not take medicines.

The Useful Family Herbal, 1754

☞ Lettuce is well known as a soporific, but it is a little startling to see it described as an opiate, which is usually defined as a drug containing or derived from opium.

For one that hath a great heat in his temples, or that cannot sleep

Take the juice of houseleek, and lettuce, of each one spoonful, of woman's milk six spoonfuls, put them together, and set them upon a chasingdish of coals, and put thereto a piece of rose-cake, and lay it to your temples.

A Choice Manual of Rare and Select Secrets in Physick and Chyrurgery, Elizabeth Grey, 1653

☞ 'Rose-cake' was rose-petals compressed to a solid lump, used primarily for perfuming linen drawers. Woman's milk may have been less easy to get hold of.

To procure sleep

Bruise a handful of aniseeds, and steep them in red rosewater, and make it up in little bags, and bind one of them to each nostril, and it will cause sleep.

The Queens Closet Opened, W.M., 1696

🖙 This would have to be very effective to overcome the annoyance of having two bags tied to your face.

For the nightmare

Item, 10 or 12 seeds of peony beaten with wine and then drunk avoid the disease called Incubus, that is the Mare, which is a sickness or fantasy oppressing a man in his sleep, that [to] him [it] seemeth a great weight lie upon his body, wherefore he groaneth and sigheth but cannot speak. If thou wilt gather again the scattered wits, then take a great basin, set it sedelings to a wall [i.e. with its side against a wall], so that it do lean wholly upon the wall; then take a laver with a cock [vessel with a tap] full of water, set it high upon a cupboard or other thing, open the cock a little so that the water drop by little and little upon the basin and make a ringing and runn out of the basin again. Into this chamber or place lay the patient so that he cannot see this nor let much be spoken to him; then doth he muse and fantasise so much upon the dropping & ringing what it may be, willing gladly to know what it is, that at the last he fasteneth his wits and gathereth them again.

A Most Excellent and Perfect Homish Apothecarye, John Hollybush's translation of Hieronymus Braunschweig, 1561

🖙 An ingenious solution to the misery of nightmares, but probably not one that would lead to calm sleep.

Gammy legs
and poor old feet

For those who could afford pattens, which lifted the wearer above the street-filth, some of the effects of poor urban drainage in pre-modern times could be avoided. Those less fortunate would have had to walk through mud and worse in worn, ill-fitting or broken shoes, with infections inevitably afflicting the feet.

For aches and swellings of the knees

Take a quart of Malmesey wine and a handful of thyme, boil them together a good space, and when it is half boiled put into it a good piece of new fresh butter, and let them boil together from a quart to a pint; and when you go to bed, bathe your knees therewith, and wet a cloth three or four times double therein, and lay it to your knees as hot as possibly you can suffer it. And so let it continue all night, and in this sort let him use this five or seven times, and doubtless it will help you. This hath been well proved.

A Rich Storehouse, or Treasurie for the Diseased, 1607

☞ Probably the warmth gave comfort. We would still use a vegetable treatment with extreme temperature, though now more likely in the form of a bag of frozen peas.

For kibed heels

Take gum dragant and galbanum, of each a like, and make thereof a powder, then take ox tallow and a little oil of violets, and melt them on the fire, and therein put the said powders, and make hereof an ointment, and herewith dress your heels.

The Widdowes Treasure, 1639

🖙 A 'kibe' was an ulcerated chilblain. 'Gum dragant and galbanum' were vegetable gums; the first was tragacanth, a traditional treatment for burns, and the second a longstanding medicinal gum, used by Hippocrates and Pliny.

Inflammation of the foot

The lungs [of a lamb] preserve the feet from inflammation occasioned by the shoes.

The History of Animals as They are Useful in Physick and Chirurgery, John Schroder, 1659

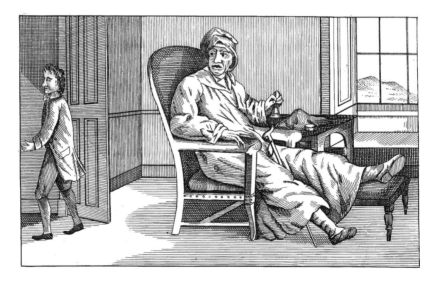

☞ The recipe does not say how the lungs are to be applied: rubbed on the feet, boiled down and applied as an embrocation, or perhaps worn as a kind of sock?

For the great oozing foot disease, which doctors call podagra

The foot is swollen and it oozes matter and pus and the sinews are contracted and the toes shrivel up. Take groundsel, that which grows in buildings, and the red 'wudufille', an equal amount of both: pound with the old fat of a pig: make it into a poultice: put on the feet: bind with a cloth over night: and wash it again in the morning and dry with a cloth: anoint with the white of a hen's egg; afterwards make a fresh poultice; do so for seven nights: then the sinews will be straight and the feet well.

The Lacnunga, eleventh century

☞ The observation of the symptoms is clear, and the frequent and regular changing of the dressing is impressive. Groundsel, cooling and antiscorbutic (effective against scurvy), was long used as a treatment for gout, which appears to be the condition described by 'podagra'. Sadly, the identification of 'wudufille' has been lost.

How to clear your feet from sweat

Take filings of pins, otherwise called pin-dust, put a little thereof into your shoes or boots, and it will keep your feet clear from sweat.

A Precious Treasury of Twenty Rare Secrets, Edward Fountaine, 1649

☞ Edward Fountaine described himself as an 'expert operator'. The filings of pins would be iron filings; the possibility of fine splinters must have made this potentially very unpleasant.

For to kill a corn

Take of the bigness of a walnut of ale yeast that is hard, and sticks to the tubside, put to it a little dried salt, finely powdered; work them well together, and put this composition into a close box; make a plaster of some of it, and bind it to the corn.

Economy of the Hands and Feet, Fingers and Toes,
'An Old Army Surgeon', 1830

☞ Brewer's yeast is one of the oldest remedies for getting rid of corns.

An excellent good remedy to take away corns in the feet or toes

First pare away the corn, and then take a black snail, and bruise it, and put a drop or two of the juice thereof into the place grieved, and put thereto a little powder of sandphere, and it will take away the corn very speedily.

A Rich Storehouse, or Treasurie for the Diseased, 1607

☞ 'Sandphere' is conceivably samphire; not generally used as an external medicinal plant, but its aroma may have been desirable here.

NERVES

THE TERM 'nerves' to mean the transmitters of sense around the body has been in use for many centuries, and the idea of 'nervous diseases' has been around since the seventeenth century.

Sage

The leaves and flowers are used as good for all diseases of the head and nerves. They are much used in all sorts of fevers, in tea or posset drink.

A Curious Herbal, Elizabeth Blackwell, 1737

🙠 Widely considered a panacea, sage has historically been linked with nervous and mental disorders.

Vertigo and falling sickness

Take the root of wild valerian and mistletoe of oak, of each an ounce; of syrup of sugar, enough to make an electuary. This is appropriated to the heart and nerves, and is good against convulsions, the vertigo and falling-sickness. The dose is the size of a walnut three times a day.

The Gentleman's, Traveller's, Husbandman and Gardener's Pocket Companion, 1751

🙠 This syrup would have been sedative from the valerian, while mistletoe has long been used for treating convulsions, hysteria and delirium. The dose is rather strong, so it cannot be recommended.

St Vitus's Dance

Symptoms. Convulsions of the legs, arms and head; inarticulate speech and lolling out of the tongue; drawing one leg after another, like an idiot; with variety of odd and ridiculous gestures. Chiefly affects the youthful.

Treatment. Emetics, cathartics, valerian root in large quantities; calcined zinc, bark, chalybeates, sea-bathing; electricity, millipedes, and quicksilver with sulphur, have been of use; as have orange leaves with the cold bath; blisters and bleeding, if judged necessary. If worms be the cause, give anthelmintics [medicines against intestinal worms].

A Medical Pocket Book, John Elliot, 1798

☞ St Vitus's Dance is a neurological disorder, characterized by jerky limb movements, which derives from a specific childhood streptococcal infection. In the pre-penicillin era the range of possible treatments was almost limitless – but note the large amount of sedative (valerian) recommended.

Electricity

General Faradisation is an essentially stimulating and tonic process, and is administered in various debilitating conditions in which by promoting the circulation, especially of the surface, causing muscular action, and accelerating waste and repair, it proves of the greatest service.

The patient either sits upon, or places the feet upon the large square metal plate connected with one terminal of the Faradic battery, while with a gentle current the whole surface of the trunk and limbs is gently sprayed by the operator, with a large sponge moistened with warm water, and attached to the other terminal. The current should be mild, and the séance last from five to ten minutes. The head should not as a rule be touched, but in the headaches of debility it is sometimes of service, if the operator holding the sponge in one hand gently passes his other hand, moistened with warm water, over the forehead and vertex.

General Faradism is employed in nervous exhaustion, sleeplessness, deficient circulation, hysteria, fatigue from over exertion, late hours, etc. The writer has recommended many patients accustomed to undergo physical fatigue – [such] as hunting men and others – to attach their sponge bath to one terminal of the faradic coil, and the sponge to the other, when they take their "tub" after a hard day's fatigue. The result is a luxurious freedom from weariness and stiffness, and a sense of renewed vigour and fitness for toil.

Electrotherapeutics, K.W. Millican, 1893

☞ The absence of a mention of any measuring device for the strength of current is rather alarming.

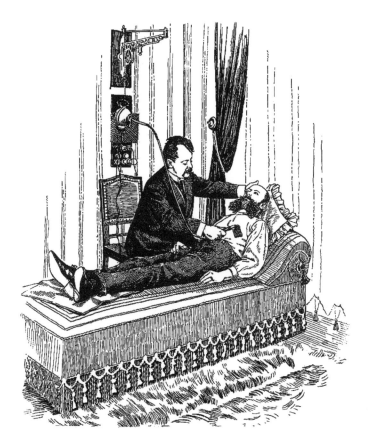

Epilepsy

The elk is a wild creature that is commonly met with in the cold
countries, especially in Sweden, Norway, Canada, and other parts …
the name Eland, or Elan, given by the Germans, signifies 'misery'; as
well because that this animal lives no where else but in desolate places,
[such] as woods, forests and the like, as because he is very subject to
the falling-sickness; and as soon as he is attacked with this disease,
he fails not to put his left foot to his left ear, to cure himself thereof;
which has given occasion to the ancients to believe that the elk's claw,
or the horn upon the left foot, was a specific for the epilepsy.

A Compleat History of Drugs, Pierre Pomet, 1737

☞ Epilepsy, having resisted all attempts at treatment, has given rise to
some desperate remedies; observation and deduction are clearly involved
in this one. A 'specific' was a remedy clearly directed at one condition or
part of the body.

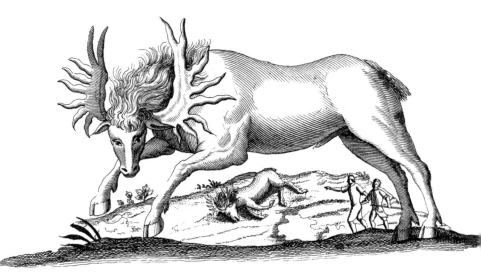

For migraine

Against pain of the head called mygrym [migraine] or cephale, give some hot opiate and the decoction of mugwort. Macer sayeth he that beareth it on him walking wearieth not. It is good against ill thoughts and stoppeth the eyes from harm and all devilishness fleeth from the place where it is.

The Great Herbal, 1526

☞ Mugwort (*Artemisia vulgaris*) was considered a wonder-herb, used for a wide range of complaints. Macer was a Roman poet who was supposed to have written a work on the virtues of herbs, but this was actually written by a medieval French physician.

Electro-therapy for nervous conditions

Directions – Connect two metallic cords or wires with the sockets in the ends of the Box, and apply the handles connected with the other ends of the metallic cords or wires to any part of the person through which it is desirable to pass the current of Electricity. Then turn the Crank, regulating the strength of the current by the speed, and by the Knob at the end of the box; it being desirable to increase the strength only to that degree most agreeable to the patient. It is less unpleasant to the patient if wet sponges are placed in the ends of the Handles, and these applied to the skin, as they prevent the pricking sensation.

Directions for Use of the Improved Magneto-electric Machine for Nervous Diseases, 1860s

☞ This kind of machine was used to treat toothache, rheumatism, tic douloureux or neuralgia, and also as a party game, with the current being passed around a circle of people holding hands. Turning the handle faster increased the amount of electricity flowing through the circuit, though there was a knob – probably controlling a resistor – to ensure that the patients were not over-stimulated.

Against the hurries

Hurries are a very disagreeable thing; they very much unfit a man either for business or company; besides, they soon degenerate into some much more serious disease: for none are stationary till they reach death. The person who is subject to hurries will find his advantage in taking the vegetable universal medicines, till such time as he finds composure, and his manner altered.

Morisoniana, James Morison, 1829

🖝 The 'hurries' was a name given to a state of agitation. In 1825 James Morison began sales of his 'vegetable pill' designed to 'purify the blood', cleverly using marketing terms that allied him to the medical profession, calling himself a 'hygeist', and establishing the British College of Health, in Bloomsbury, as a sales outlet. At the height of their success the pills were being used for most diseases (and, inevitably, snakebite), with nearly one billion sold in the decade to 1850; this figure depended largely on the dosage of twenty to thirty pills per day. Their composition was a mix of aloes, tartaric acid, senna, colocynth, gamboge, rhubarb and myrrh (so, basically, a laxative). The commercial success boosted the regard in which they were popularly held; they were still being sold, despite being heavily satirized, in the 1920s.

For the headache

It is good for the headache if the temples and the forehead be anointed with oil of roses and vinegar.

The Great Herbal, 1526

🖝 It works.

SICKNESS AND DISEASES

THE GRADUAL development of medicine over the centuries has increased the number of identified diseases. What was actually meant by 'flux' or 'consumption' in pre-modern times is often unclear, and the waters are muddied by changes in the application of such terms as 'jaundice' or 'cholera'.

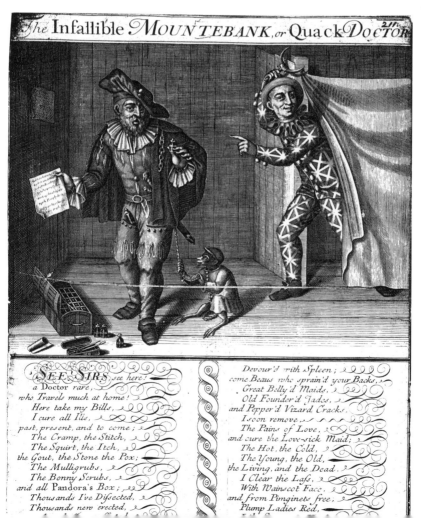

The Infallible MOUNTEBANK, or Quack Doctor

SEE SIRS, see here!
a Doctor rare,
who Travels much at home!
Here take my Bills,
I cure all Ills,
past, present, and to come;
The Cramp, the Stitch,
The Squirt, the Itch,
the Gout, the Stone the Pox;
The Mulligrubs,
The Bonny Scrubs,
and all Pandora's Box;
Thousands I've Dissected,
Thousands new erected,

Devour'd with Spleen;
come Beaus who sprain'd your Backs,
Great Belly'd Maids,
Old Founder'd Jades,
and Pepper'd Vizard Cracks.
I soon remove
The Pains of Love,
and cure the Love-sick Maid;
The Hot, the Cold,
The Young, the Old,
the Living, and the Dead.
I Clear the Lass
With Wainscot Face,
and from Pimginets free,
Plump Ladies Red,

Cock-water for consumption

Take a running cock, pull him alive, then kill him, cut him across the back, take out the entrails and wipe him clean, then quarter him and break his bones, then put him into rose-water still with a pottle of sack [sherry], currants and raisins stoned, and figs sliced, of each one pound, dates stoned, and cut small half a pound, rosemary flowers, wild thyme, spearmint, of each one handful, organs [oregano] or wild marjoram, bugloss, pimpernel, of each two handfuls, and a pottle of new milk from a red cow. Distil these with a soft fire, put into the receiver a quarter of a pound of sugarcandy beaten small, four grains of amber-greece [ambergris], forty grains of prepared pearl, and half a book of leaf gold cut very small; you must mingle the strong water with the small, and let the patient take two spoonfuls of it in the morning, and as much at going to bed.

The Queens Closet Opened, W.M., 1696

☞ The cock was plucked before dispatch, and the recipe is a mix of nutritious herbs and dried fruits; the gold-leaf was probably just an encouragement to the patient that the medicine was expensive and therefore effective. 'Pearl' here was a substance used for clarifying wine, often made from dried egg white.

Jaundice

Symptoms: yellowness of the whole skin, but chiefly the whites of the eyes; the urine also yellow; lassitude, inactivity, anxiety, sickness, oppression and difficult breathing; pain at the stomach; bitter taste in the mouth; sometimes attended with purging, at others costiveness; stools generally like blue clay, but sometimes of a dark earthy, and at others of a deep yellow colour.

Treatment: if the vessels be very full, bleed; then vomit, purge and give medicines with soap; to which may occasionally be added, rhubarb, aloes, chalybeates or squills [tubers of the sea-onion]. Saline draughts if fever; opiates in case of pain; gentle emetics may be occasionally repeated, and the body should be kept open. Chalybeate waters, or water or cider with a red hot iron quenched in it, may be used as common drink; gentle exercise, air, and company.

A Medical Pocket Book, John Elliot, 1798

☞ Anaemia-induced jaundice responds to iron supplements, here supplied by quenching red-hot iron in liquid, or iron-rich chalybeate water.

King's evil or scrofula

Take mercurius dulcis one dram, antimony revived half a dram. You may give of this medicine three, four or five grains, according to age or strength of the patient. Take this twice a week.

In the intermediate days, use the diet drink following:

Take of the leaves of senna half a pound, the root of monks rhubarb seven ounces, the roots of polypody of oak [a fern], of each four ounces, the roots of mizerion three ounces and a half, rue leaves, whitlow-grass, three handfuls, rinds of oranges dried six ounces, crude antimony grossly powdered one pound; slice and bruise these, then put them in a bag, and boil them in four gallons and a half of middling [medium-strength] drink, to three gallons. Take half a pint every morning, increasing or lessening the dose according to its operation. By this method I have cured great numbers.

The Ancient Physician's Legacy to his Country, Thomas Dover, 1733

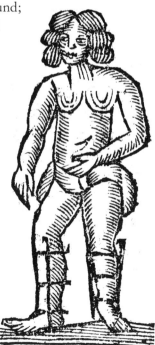

☞ Scrofula is characterized by chronic enlargement and degeneration of the lymph glands; a traditional cure was to have the patient touched by royalty, hence its other name. The real surprise here is 'mizerion' (the plant mezereon), which is highly toxic, and even at this proportionately low level, very dangerous. *Mercurius dulcis* is still used as a homeopathic remedy for dropsies.

A brief guide to the common people of New England how to order themselves and theirs in the small-pocks or measels

Before the fourth day use no medicines to drive out, nor be too strict with the sick; for by how much the more gently the pustules do grow, by so much the fuller and perfecter will the separation be.

On the fourth day a gentle cordial may help once.

From that time a small draught of warm milk (not hot) a little dyed with saffron may be given morning and evening till the pustules are come to their due greatness and ripeness.

When the pustules begin to dry and crust, lest the rotten vapours strike inward, which sometimes causeth sudden death, take morning and evening some temperate cordial, as four or five spoonfuls of malaga wine tinged with a little saffron.

When the pustules are dry and fallen off, purge once and again, especially in the autumn pox.

Beware of anointing with oils, fats, ointments, and such defensives, for keeping the corrupted matter in the pustules from drying up; by the moisture they fret deeper into the flesh, and so make the more deep scars.

Deadly signs: if the flux of the belly happen, when they are broke forth, if the urine be bloody, or black, or the ordure of that colour; or if pure blood be cast out by the belly or gums; these signs are for the most part deadly.

Thomas Thacher, 1678

☞ The text is notable for its calm tone and general good sense. Thacher describes himself at the end of this pamphlet as 'no physitian, yet a well wisher to the sick', and indeed he is careful to point out that his advice is for those who cannot get to a doctor. He goes out of his way not to offend 'the Learned Physitian, that hath much more cause to understand what pertains to this disease than I'.

Syrup of hartstongue

Take of polipodium of the oak [a fern], the roots of both sorts of Bugloss, bark of capparoots [possibly caper], bark of tamarisk, of each two ounces, hartstongue three handfuls, hops, dodder, maiden-hair, balm of each two handfuls; boil them in nine pints of water, till there remains but five, strain it, clarify it, and with four pound of white sugar boil it into a syrup.

It opens obstructions of the liver and spleen, and is profitable against splenetic evils, and is therefore a choice remedy [for that] which the vulgar call the rickets, or liver-grown; a spoonful in a morning is a precious remedy for children troubled with that disease. Men that are troubled with the spleen, which is known by pain and hardness in their left side, may take three or four spoonfuls; they shall find this one receipt worth the price of the whole book.

A Physical Directory, Nicholas Culpeper, 1651

 Rickets was thought of as a new disease at this time, and Culpeper was one of its early investigators, hence his concern to separate it from other conditions. Hart's tongue (a fern) taken as an infusion is still used to treat blood-flow obstructions in the liver and spleen.

Phenitis or inflammation of the brain

In an inflammation of the brain, nothing more certainly relieves the patient than a free discharge of blood from the nose. When this comes of its own accord it is by no means to be stopped, but promoted, by applying cloths dipped in warm water to the part. When bleeding at the nose does not happen spontaneously, it may be provoked, by putting a straw, or any other sharp object, up the nostril.

Domestic Medicine, William Buchan, 1774

☞ Buchan was a great believer in the curative power of bleeding; the term 'phenitis' has been superseded by meningitis.

A medicine to drive out the small pox

Take milk, saffron and English honey, and seethe them together and give it to the patient and let him be kept warm, and this will bring forth the pox in a short space.

A Rich Storehouse, or Treasurie for the Diseased, 1607

☞ Treatment here is concentrated on the manifestation of the disease by the pustules appearing, though it would have been identified by the body rash and, before that, the sores in the mouth; this recipe was probably aimed at soothing the discomfort of the mouth sores.

A gargarism against the scurvy

Rosemary 1 handful, cloves 40, salt of scurvy-grass 2 oz, omphacine 3 lb; boil to 2 lb. It is good for putrid gums in the scurvy.

Bates' Dispensatory, translated and edited by William Salmon, 1694

☞ A 'gargarism' is a gargle. Salmon states that 'If the gums be putrefied, or cankers be present in them, it must be often used in a day at least five or six times, till it is apparent that the putrefaction is mastered. After that you may gargle with white-wine wherein a little salt of scurvy-grass is dissolved.'

Long before the introduction of lemons and limes into the diets of sailors, scurvy-grass was a welcome food for returning mariners. It grows widely in coastal areas in the northern hemisphere, and is rich in Vitamin C.

Of the apoplexy

It consists in a most profound sleep, and total privation of sense and motion, excepting only respiration, which is still performed, but with difficulty and snoring.

Let a vein be instantly opened in the arm, and twelve ounces of blood taken away and afterwards eight ounces more out of the jugulars. Immediately after exhibit [give] a vomit of an ounce and a half, or two ounces of the infusion of Crocus Metallorum.

Let a large and sharp blistering plaster be applied to the hinder part of the neck.

While these things are doing, let the sick person sit upright in his bed, not oppressed with too great a burden of clothes.

Let spirit of Sal Armoniac, excellently rectified, be held to his nose.

The Compleat Method of Curing Almost All Diseases, Thomas Sydenham, 1694

🖙 An apoplexy is a failure of neurological functions due to cerebral haemorrhage. Taking blood from the arm and, alarmingly, the jugular veins would be intended to relieve the head of too much blood.

For a bruise in a woman's breast that is hard, swollen

Take woodlice, and dry them between papers before the fire, and make them into fine powder, whereof take as much as will lie on a threepence in a spoonful of grout ale; do this first and last for three weeks together, and after you may take twice a week till you find the breast well. But you must be sure to keep a white cotton fried in goose-grease to it constantly, though you leave taking the powder, until you find the breast cured. This hath cured the breasts that should have been cut off.

The Queens Closet Opened, W.M., 1696

🖙 This appears to be breast cancer; the reference to mastectomy indicates that it was taken very seriously. An alternative to mastectomy – the novelist Fanny Burney underwent the operation without anaesthetic in 1810 – would have been much appreciated.

Cancer

Take a white oak root and bore out the heart and burn the chips to get the ashes, ¼ oz; lunar caustic ¼ oz; calomel ¼ oz; saltpetre ¼ oz; all to be made fine and mixed with ¼ lb of lard.

Spread this thin upon soft leather and apply it to the cancer, changing it twice a day; it will kill the tumor in 3–4 days; which you will know by the general appearance; then apply a poultice of soaked figs until it comes out, fibres and all; heal with a plaster made by boiling red beech leaves in water, straining and boiling thick; then mix with bees' wax and mutton tallow to form a salve of proper consistency. To cleanse the system ensure the above is being used and for some time after.

The Book You Want: How to Cure Everything, How to Do Everything, Receipts for Everything, John King, 1885

☛ This is L.S. Hodgkin's method, from Reding, Michigan, for cancer of the breast: he cured his wife. Other quoted 'cures' involved yellow dock root, used as a tea and poultice (Ohio); red clover, poke (possibly *Nicotiana rustica*) and yellow-dock (Philadelphia, Professor Calkins); and red oak bark (John Dillon of Zanesville).

A vulgar error

That Abracadabra written on a piece of paper, worn on the stomach will in a few days effectively cure a jaundice.

When the jaundice has been caused by grumous concretions of bile stopping up its passage from the gall bladder; the bile, by filling the bladder, may, after a little time, by its distension, force out the stone that stopped it, and thus give Abracadabra the credit of the cure.

Medical, Philosophical and Vulgar Errors of Various Kinds Considered and Refuted, John Jones, 1797

☛ Jones proposes correctly that thick bile becoming crystallized into gallstones can block the common bile duct, causing jaundice; conceivably pressure could force a gallstone out, but Jones is understandably annoyed that credit for the expulsion of the stones should be given to a charm.

Marasmus and diarrhoea

Mr J R of Ho— Ohio, merchant, of slender habit, and light complexion, aged 30 years. Called to see him November 5th 1833. He has tubercles and ulcers on both sides of the neck, the tubercles very large, and has also an enlargement of the abdomen, with irregular fever and diarrhoea, and is pale and much emaciated.

The disease commenced a few months since after an attack of bilious fever. Diagnosis: Tubercula of the neck, intestines, and mesentery. Prescribed Elecro-Magnetic pills and plaster. His fever and diarrhoea disappeared in a few days, and his health soon began to improve, and in six weeks he was restored, and has gained during this time considerable flesh and strength.

These remedies are a preparation of gold, made and maintained in a negative state, and put up in the form of pills; and a preparation of iron, made and maintained in a positive state, and put up in the form of a plaster. That is, the pills received a negative charge, and the plaster a positive charge.

*Electro-Galvanic Symptoms and Electro-Magnetic
Remedies*, H.H. Sherwood, 1837, New York

☞ 'Marasmus', a term meaning any wasting disease, had been abandoned by *The Lancet* by this time, as more specific diseases were being defined. The 'mesentery' was at this time the membrane supporting the viscera within the abdomen.

For the bloody flux

The bramble, or black-berry-bush. The flowers and fruit unripe are very binding, and so profitable for the bloody flux, lasks, and are a fit remedy for spitting of blood.

Balm. It is good to wash aching teeth therewith, and profitable for those that have the bloody flux.

Agrimony. The leaves and seed taken in wine, stayeth the bloody flux.

Golden Rod. The decoction of the herb green or dry, or the distilled water thereof is very effectual for inward bruises, as also to be outwardly applied, it stayeth bleeding in any part of the body, and of wounds also, the fluxes of humours, the bloody flux, and women's courses.

The English Physitian, Nicholas Culpeper, 1652

☞ Dysentery (the 'bloody flux') was endemic in early-modern society in which the rapid growth of cities and towns led to dense living conditions with poor clean water supplies, little sewage management and limited domestic sanitation; armies on the march suffered greatly. Hence the proliferation of treatments for the condition.

'England's Solar Pill against the Scurvy'

This noble solar pill cures that inveterate disease the scurvy, with all its symptoms, which are pains in the head, inflammations in the brain, frenzies, madness, megrims, convulsions, falling sickness, tremblings and weakness of the limbs, etc [the list runs to over 40] nay, the plague itself is but a high graduated scurvy, as appeared in our last great plague; for nothing was then found effectual for prevention or cure, but pure and high exalted antiscorbutics.

Quack's handbill, *c*.1700

☞ Identifying the disease by a cure is an interesting process; the list of symptoms claimed for scurvy is impressive too. 'Solar' medicines, in various forms, claimed to harness the power of sunbeams: there were also solar tinctures, which claimed to be able to provide 'Relief and Comfort to all Mankind'.

Sore eyes

The dust and draughts of pre-modern buildings were a major cause of eye infections; many poor people would have slept on the floor. Rush coverings of medieval floors, renewed infrequently, would have harboured many sources of infection. Remedies for eye infections feature widely in pre-modern medical compendiums.

The removal of a cataract

A cataract can only be treated by handy work, and to do that, it is needful a surgeon do first learn, and see it done, of a cunning man that can well remove, and put it away; [it is done] with an instrument made like a needle, which must be pressed into the coniunctiva, fixing it inward transversely, till the needle (which the workman shall still behold, as it passeth under the cornea), shall come to the water, which is placed before the hole of the pupilla, which doth prohibit the sight. And then thou mayest put it down till the patient may see; and after that put him 10 days in a dark house, in silence, without noise, and bind upon the eye an emplaster of *bole armenio distemperato cum albumine ovi* [Armenian clay with egg white], put between two pieces of linen cloth.

Chirurgerie, John Hall's translation of Lanfranc, 1565

☞ Cataracts have been treated as removable for several centuries: in this step-by-step guide the job is done by a surgeon, of a lower status than a physician, who limited his role to observing and prescribing. The use of egg white, reminiscent of the first aid given to Gloucester after his blinding in Shakespeare's *King Lear*, may have been largely based on the similarity of texture to that of the liquids inside the eye. The Armenian clay acted as an astringent, which would contract the tissue and help healing.

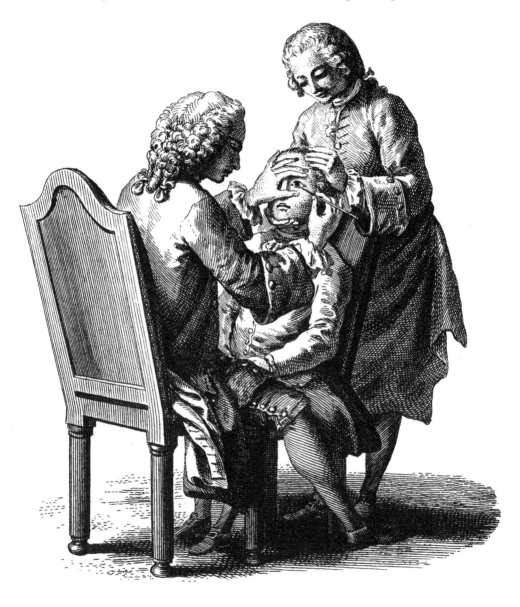

Eyes web

Mire doves' dung with vinegar, and apply it.

The Garden of Health, William Langham, 1578

🖙 Langham's use of bird droppings in the eyes was continued into the eighteenth century by, among others, Sir William Read, oculist to Queen Anne, whose treatment involved 'the juice of goose dung or the white part of hen's dung'. The main constituents of hen dung are nitrogen, phosphorus and potassium, with a wide range of traces of other minerals, but the near-certainty of transmitting disease through fungal infection must have outweighed any possible benefits.

Electro therapeutics of the eye

For neuralgic, rheumatic, or painful affections of, or about the eye, the Faradaic current must be used, or is to be preferred; but where stimulation of the optic nerve is required, then we may use frictional electricity. Negative sparks may be drawn from the eyeball through the closed eyelid; or galvanisation may be used, by applying the positive sponge electrode over the affected eye, and the negative applied to the nape of the neck; or both conductors may be applied to the nape of the neck; or both conductors may be applied to each closed eye, for a few seconds only at a time. Flashes of light, or a metallic taste, will be sufficient evidence that the current is strong enough.

The Practice of Medical Electricity, George Powell, 1869

🖙 Faradaic current is inductive, that is current caused by placing the conductor in a changing magnetic field, while frictional current is produced by rubbing, and galvanization is produced from a battery, through a chemical reaction. All of them, applied to the eye, sound worrying.

Some Anglo-Saxon treatments for swollen eyes

Take a living raven, take the eyes out of it and, still living, bring it into water, and put the eyes on the neck of the man to whom they are needful, and he will soon be hale. Make a good eye-salve. Take celandine and bishopwort, wormwood, woodparsley, woodbine's leaf, put equal amounts of all, crush them well, put them into honey and wine; and put two-thirds of the wine and a third of the honey into a brass or copper vessel so that the liquid will be able to cover the plants, moreover; let it stand for seven nights and cover with a board, strain the drink through a clean cloth, put it back in the same vessel, use it as may be needful to you.

For swollen eyes, take a live crab, remove the eyes, and afterwards put it alive into the water, and hang the eyes around the neck of anyone who has need of them.

To make an eye salve for a stye: take an onion and garlic equal amounts of both, pound well together, take wine and bull's gall equal amounts of both, mix with the leeks, them put in a brass vessel, let stand for nine nights in the brass vessel, strain through a cloth and clear well, put in a horn and about night time put on the eye with a feather, the best remedy.

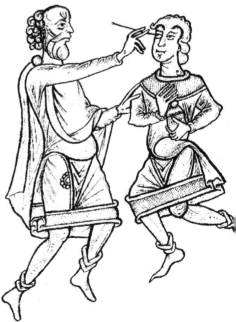

Medicines for dimness of the eyes; take the juice or blossoms of celandine, mix with bumblebees' honey, put in a brass vessel, make lukewarm skilfully over warm coals until it is cooked.

☞ As M.L. Cameron has shown, Anglo-Saxon remedies often contained ingredients which would have been effective, despite the absence of modern scientific processes. The onion and garlic in the third recipe would have provided an antibiotic against staphylococcal infection, ox gall would have worked against bacteria, the wine would have produced cytotoxic acetates and tartarates, and the copper part of the brass would have produced bactericidal copper salts, long known to be a defence against eye infections.

The fourth recipe uses celandine, long used in treatments for eye infections; the plant gives off a bright orange latex when it is broken. In its raw state this is an irritant, but when warmed it is an effective treatment against film or spots on the surface of the eye. The honey used in many of the recipes acted as a bactericide, and is often specified as bumblebee honey, probably due to a scribe's mistake in copying 'Atticus [Greek] honey' as 'Attacus [wild insect] honey' – bumblebees are the only wild insects in Britain that produce enough honey to be harvestable. Note how the reader is warned not to boil the liquid.

A treatment for an eye-injury

There was a boy from Tiverton in Devon about 12 years of age who lost the sight of one eye after a blow to it, so that he could not see at all with the other eye closed. Twice daily I put in the affected eye swallow's blood, and he drank daily betony mashed up with ale, and within fifteen days he had recovered his sight by the grace of God. And certainly in many cases I have discovered betony to be effective in getting rid of all fleshy growths in the eyes when drunk in this fashion, and after bathing with rosewater or similar.

Commonplace Book and Medical Miscellany,
Thomas Fayreford, fifteenth century

☞ Why swallow's blood? It cannot have been easy to acquire, other than from nestlings; it was believed that eating a swallow's heart brought increased memory and intelligence, but the connection to sight may have been a very localized tradition. And besides, Fayreford seems more interested in the healing power of betony.

Treatment for ophthalmia or inflammation of the eyes

Bleeding, in a violent inflammation of the eyes, is always necessary. This should be performed as near the part affected as possible. An adult may lose ten or twelve ounces of blood from the jugular vein, and the operation may be repeated according to the urgency of the symptoms. If it should not be convenient to bleed in the neck, the same quantity may be let from the arm, or any other part of the body.

Leeches are often applied to the temples, or under the eyes, with good effect. The wounds must be suffered to bleed for some hours and if the bleeding stop soon, it may be promoted by the application of cloths dipt in warm water. In obstinate cases, it will be necessary to repeat this operation several times.

When the disease has been of long standing, I have seen very extraordinary effects from a seton in the neck, or between the shoulders, especially the latter. It should be upwards and downwards, or in the direction of the spine, and in the middle between the shoulder blades. It may be dressed twice a day with ointment of yellow wax [yellow basilicon ointment]. I have known patients, who had been blind for a considerable time, recover sight by means of a seton placed as above. When the seton is put across the neck, it soon wears out, and is both more painful and troublesome than between the shoulders; besides, it leaves a disagreeable mark, and does not discharge so freely.

Domestic Medicine, William Buchan, 1830

🖙 Buchan (or later editors of the book credited to him, which remained in print for over sixty years) proposed that ophthalmia, or inflammation of the eyes, was 'often caused by the stoppage of the customary evacuations' (constipation and so on) and other curious causes, such as 'the suppressing of gentle morning sweats', as well as more obvious circumstances such as exposure to smoke.

Aches and pains, colds and fevers

IT should not be thought that the only pain-relievers in pre-modern times were brandy and/or chewing on leather. White-willow bark (a source of salicylic acid, a constituent of aspirin), belladonna, arnica, fennel seeds, feverfew and many others were all available, and many of them are still in use.

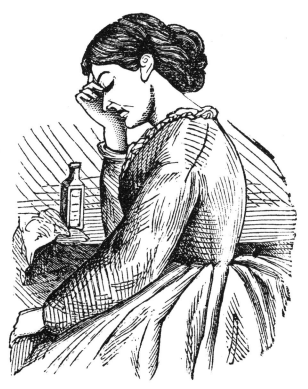

Neck pain

For neck pain boil the lower part of nettle in ox's grease and in butter, then smear the thigh for neck pain, and if the thigh should be painful smear the neck with the salve. Again, boil the lower part of nettle in vinegar, put ox's gall in the vinegar and take the plant out, smear the neck with it.

Bald's Leechbook, Anglo-Saxon manuscript

☞ This looks almost to be using the principles of acupuncture or reflexology, particularly the perceived sympathy between different parts of the body. Either way, nettle used with fat and vinegar is a traditional treatment for muscular pain.

A present remedy for an old ache

Take very strong aquavitae, and two spoonfuls of the water of arstmart, and annoint the place where the ache is, every day two or three times, and it will speedily heal it.

A Rich Storehouse, or Treasurie for the Diseased, 1607

☞ 'Arstmart', or more usually 'arsesmart', was water pepper, a plant which irritated sensitive skin; it has been used to treat a wide range of complaints, from coughs to rheumatism. 'Aquavitae' here was unrefined alcohol rather than a strong drink.

Oil of foxes, or badgers, for ache in the joints, the sciatica, diseases of the sinews, and pains of the reins and back

Take a live fox, or badger, of a middle age, well fed, and fat; kill him, bowel [gut] him, and skin him; some take out his bowels, but some only his excrements in his guts, because his guts have much grease about them; break his bones small that you may have all the marrow; this done, set him boiling in salt brine, and seawater, and salt water, of each a pint and half, of oil three pints, of salt three ounces; in the end of decoction put thereto the leaves of sage, rosemary, dill, oregano, marjoram, and juniper berries, and when he is so sodden as that his bones and flesh do part in sunder, strain all through a strainer, and keep it in a vessel to make linaments for the ache in the joints, the sciatica, diseases of the sinews, and pains of the reins and back.

A Choice Manual of Rare and Select Secrets in Physick and Chyrurgery, Elizabeth Grey, 1653

☞ There was little room for sentiment towards animals during the mid-seventeenth century. But why the three types of salt water? And would there really be no difference between using a fox and a badger?

Against a side-ache

Betony, bishopwort, elecampane, radish, the sorrel which may float, horehound, groundsel, cropleek, garlic, rue, hindhealth, lupin, horehound; boil in butter; smear the sides with it; he will be better.

The Lacnunga, eleventh century

☞ Variously identified as vervain or marshmallow, 'bishopwort' appears in another text in a recipe for aching thighs; vervain is a wonder-herb, with claims to be able to heal conditions as various as epilepsy, myopia and dysentery. 'Hindhealth' is connected to deer, and may be sage-leaved germander or tansy (also known as 'hindheal'), which improves the circulation and is used to treat bruises and varicose veins.

The various useful properties of the water of alchimilla or lions foot

A dram of the powder of it, taken with three ounces of the water, helpeth the falling of the bowels into the cod, or other rupture in short time, without any cutting.

The Newe Jewell of Health, George Baker's translation of Conrad Gessner, 1576

☞ This sounds like a prolapsed rectum. *Alchemilla mollis* (Lady's mantle) was thought to have the ability to tighten and reinvigorate flagging parts of the body.

Of centumpedes, call'd in English 'sows'

If you minister the powder of these creatures in wine it hath many excellent properties, but chiefly it hath been experienced greatly to prevail against the stitch in the side, for it will help that grief presently.

Polypharmakos, Daniel Border, 1651

🖝 Rather than centipedes, 'sows' were millipedes, or more often woodlice, regularly used in medicine well into the eighteenth century.

The palsy tincture

Powder of cantharides, bishopsweed, spirit of wine rectified, mix, and extract a tincture, which strain. It is to be rubbed upon the paralytic members.

The intention of this medicine is only for friction, which is so often to be repeated, till the part grows red and, in some thin skinned people, is blistered; till blisters arise you may use it twice a day, or oftener; for by this means the animal spirits are attracted into this part, and the natural heat is revived.

Bates' Dispensatory, translated and edited by William Salmon, 1694

🖝 A palsy here is a paralysis or weakness of a part of the body, in which the surface circulation would be stimulated by friction with the additional stimulant of cantharides – also known as Spanish Fly – a powder of dried beetles, which caused blisters and made the skin red.

For sprains, strains, lame back and rheumatism

Good sized live toads, four in number: put into boiling water and cook very soft; then take them out and boil the water down to ½ pint, and add fresh churned, unsalted butter 1 lb and simmer together; at the last add tincture of arnica 2 oz.

This was obtained from an old physician, who thought more of it than of any other prescription in his possession. Some persons might think it hard on toads, but you could not kill them quicker in any other way.

The Book You Want: How to Cure Everything, How to Do Everything, Receipts for Everything, John King 1885

🙠 John King's book of remedies collected from around the USA included several folk recipes that look decidedly out of date for 1885, the year in which Pasteur successfully tested his vaccine against rabies. Over the centuries amphibians have had good cause for protest against Western medicine.

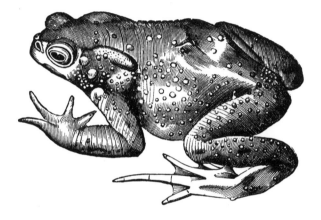

For rhumatics

One penny-worth of hartshorn, one raw egg well beaten, half pint vinegar, one ounce spirits of turpentine, quarter ounce spirits of wine, quarter ounce of camphor, beaten well together ten minutes. Cork down tightly; in half an hour fit for use.

The New Practical Family Physician, Thomas Churchill, 1808

🙠 This was found as a handwritten note in a copy of the book, along with small handbills for Wand's Bowel Complaint Mixture, George Wilby's Aromatic Steel Pills, Hall's 'Lung Restorer' and others. A testimonial quoted in a handbill for 'Poor Richard's Stomach Pills' is dated 1843, showing that this book was in use for at least thirty-five years.

For inflammation

If the inflammation should be permanent in one place, make a good bathing; take ivy which grows on a stone on the earth, and yarrow and woodbine's leaf, and cowslip and oxlip; pound them all very well; lay them on a hot stone in a trough, put a little water in, let it steam on the body, as much as may be needful for him, until it be cool; put another hot stone in; bathe often, soon better will be for him.

The Lacnunga, eleventh century

☛ The warm bath with infusions of herbs sounds enticing, and this recipe shows that it could be achieved fairly easily.

Plaster for the feet in fevers

Take of galbanum half an ounce, burgundy pitch half an ounce, mix and apply spread on linen, over both the feet, in fevers where there is too great a circulation towards the head; this will give relief.

The Family Physician, Edward Bullman, 1789

☛ The idea here is that the cold material would draw heat towards the feet, away from the head.

Fumigation for fevers

In situations where the constitution of the air renders these fevers very common, the inhabitants should frequently burn in their rooms, at least in their lodging rooms, some aromatic wood or herbs. They should daily chew some juniper-berries, and drink a fermented infusion of them. These two remedies are very effectual to fortify the weakest stomachs, to prevent obstructions, and to promote perspiration. And, as these are the causes which prolong these fevers the most obstinately, nothing is a more certain preservation from them than these cheap and obvious assistances.

Advice to People in General with Respect to their Health,
Samuel Tissot, translated by 'A Physician', 1766

A century after the Great Plague physicians still believed that disease in enclosed spaces could be prevented by fumigation of the air itself. A fermented infusion of juniper berries is, more or less, gin.

A very good drink for the voiding of phlegm, and for the stopping of the pipes

Take a pot of barley, and seethe it in a gallon of well-water, and let it seethe until the barley be lost; then strain it and put thereto as much new wort as of the aforesaid licquor, and put therein a good quantity of sage, and as much hyssop, and a pennyworth of liquorice well bruised; then seethe it again until it be half consumed away; then strain it and put it into a glass, or into some other close vessel, and so let it stand the space of one whole day, and let the party grieved drink two or three spoonfuls of it at a time, both morning and evening, and this will help him in a short space. This hath been well proved.

A Rich Storehouse, or Treasurie for the Diseased, 1607

'Wort' is unfermented beer – the mix of grain and water, which would be soothing to drink; hyssop is a good expectorant, while sage has long been used against fevers. Liquorice's soothing properties mean that it is still a common ingredient in cough medicines.

CHILDREN

U NTIL the late nineteenth century, infant mortality was so high that to many parents it must have seemed that babies were 'on loan'. And even after infancy they were all too susceptible to diseases such as 'chincough' (whooping cough) or 'squinancy' (quinsy).

Teething

Most infants breed their teeth with pain, and numbers die at that period, particularly in cutting their canines, or eye teeth, which have their origin near the nerves, which pass by the eyes, and are very irritable in young children, causing convulsions, severe gangrene, excessive purging, etc. I have found the anodyne necklace the most safe and efficacious remedy that can be used, and to administer gentle purges in case of costiveness, such as senna and prunes stewed; manna, magnesia, and rhubarb mixed, according to the age of the child – The diet should be light and nourishing.

Anodyne necklace – take henbane root, dry it, and cut it into small round beads, string them on silk, and steep in a little spirits of lavender to give it a little colour; when dry tie it around the child's neck, and let it remain till all the teeth are cut through the gums.

The Family Physician, Edward Bullman, 1789

☞ As so many children succumbed to diseases just as they were beginning to teethe, and as relief of teething pain often caused them to stop crying, it was natural to believe that children died from teething, and that teething was related to more serious conditions. Hence the proliferation of treatments, some of them wild and desperate, others apparently simple and reasonable, for sore gums in infancy. Tying anything around a young child's neck would set parental alarm bells ringing now.

To make children's teeth come without pain. Proved

Take the head of a hare boiled or roasted, and with the brains thereof mingle honey and butter, and therewith anoint the child's gums as often as you please.

The Queens Closet Opened, W.M., 1696

☞ This may be a local or family recipe; I can find no reason why, specifically, a hare should be used. Its flesh was considered a 'melancholy meat' within the Galenic system.

Powder to kill worms

Take the child's own hair, cut it small, so as to appear like powder, as much as will lay on a silver penny, mix it with honey or treacle, adding to each dose half a grain of hellebore. Give three mornings together, fasting three days before the full of the moon, and repeat it till the worms are destroyed.

The Family Physician, Edward Bullman, 1789

☞ At times Bullman's advice seems quite sensible; at others it is bizarre. Hellebore is a powerful emetic and purgative, but very dangerous.

Of the scarlet fever

Children are chiefly infected with it about the latter end of summer. At the first they are seized with a coldness and shivering, yet they are not very sick. The whole skin is spotted with little red specks, that are thicker, broader, and of a redder colour than in the measles. They continue two or three days, and then disappear, and the upmost skin falling off, that which is under it appears stained with measly scales.

Take burnt hartshorn and compound powder of crabs-claws, of each half a dram; cochineal two grains; sugar-candy one dram; mix them, and beat them to a very fine powder, to be divided into twelve papers, of which one is to be taken every sixth hour, drinking after them two or three spoonfuls of the following julep.

Take black-cherry water, milkwater, of each three ounces; syrup of the juice of citrons one ounce; mix them and make a julep.

Let a blistering plaster be also applied to the hinder part of the neck, and every night exhibit a composing draught of syrup of meconium [an opiate]; and the symptoms ceasing, prescribe a purging medicine.

The Compleat Method of Curing Almost All Diseases, Thomas Sydenham, 1694

🖙 This recipe includes three of Sydenham's regular favourites: 'black-cherry water', made from the bark of the black or wild cherry, a 'julep' (sweet drink), and a purge to finish with. Of interest also is the direction to divide the medicine into 'papers', indicating how it would be stored ready for use against this killer disease.

A medicine for a child that cannot hold his or her water

Take the navel-string of a child, which is ready to fall from him, dry it and beat it to powder, and give it to the patient child male or female in two spoonfuls of small beer to drink fasting in the morning.

The Queens Closet Opened, W.M., 1696

🖙 This treatment for incontinence defies any attempt at rational explanation.

Rickets

This disease proceeds from a relaxed habit, after illness, or from bad nursing; therefore the cure must be performed by diet of a strengthening nature, good air, and plenty of exercise, avoiding weak watery things, especially tea; the cold bath is of infinite service to those who have it brought on by illness, also the peruvian bark; which may be given to two drams a day, in any form the child will take it. Those who do not approve of the cold bath may wash the child all over in cold water every morning, and rub it dry with a coarse cloth.

To children of a gross habit gentle purges of rhubarb may be given frequently.

The Family Physician, Edward Bullman, 1789

An outbreak of disease in the seventeenth century led to the identification of rickets, thenceforth called 'the English disease', but it was work on vitamins that proved that rickets was specifically a vitamin- and nutrition-deficiency disease. The references to diet and exercise in this remedy may have helped, though cold baths and purges are indicative of standard treatments that would have little efficacy compared to a good dose of sunlight. Peruvian bark was chinchona, the source of quinine, while 'gross habit' here seems to be self-induced constipation.

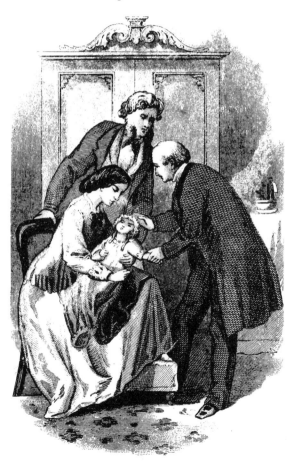

Godfrey's Cordial

As our German peasants are cupped and bled at certain seasons, so do the English working people now consume patent medicines to their own injury and to the great profit of the manufacturer. One of the most injurious of these patent medicines is a drink prepared with opiates, chiefly laudanum, under the name Godfrey's Cordial. Women who work at home, and who have their own and other people's children to take care of, give them this drink to keep them quiet, and, as many believe, to strengthen them. They often begin to give this medicine to newly-born children and continue, without knowing the effect of this 'heartsease', until the children die. The less susceptible the child's system to the action of the opium, the greater the quantities administered. When the cordial ceases to act, laudanum alone is given, often to the extent of fifteen to twenty drops at a dose.

The Condition of the Working Class in England
in 1844, Friedrich Engels

☞ Laudanum (effectively opium) continued to be used in patent medicines well into the twentieth century; Engels shows that increasing doses given to children were ultimately fatal.

To prevent bed-wetting

A mouse rotted and given to children to eat remedieth pissing the bed.

The Widdowes Treasure, 1639

☞ Note what is actually written: presumably the intention was a 'scare cure'. Probably, given the awfulness of some recipes around at this time, some children accepted the medicine stoically, and were very, very ill – and presumably continued to wet the bed as well.

MEDICINE CHEST

PROPRIETARY MEDICINES have been available for several centuries, and brand names contribute to our not knowing what we are using. In recent decades boracic acid tape and bottles of witch hazel have largely disappeared from the bathroom cabinet, but probably few households ever kept stocks of ostrich fat, crabs' eyes or hippopotamus skin.

To make oil of the skull of a man

Take the skull of a man that was never buried, and break it into powder, then distill away the phlegm with a gentle fire, and put it on again, and distill it again; and this you shall do three times upon the feces [residue], and at the last give it strong fire, until the oil be come forth; the which ye shall separate by Balneo [bain marie], and keep it close shut in a glass. The dose is three grains, against the falling sickness. Ye shall understand, that there is also salt to be drawn forth from the feces, which is of great virtue against the aforesaid diseases being drunk with wine.

The Secrets of Physick and Philosophy, John Hester's
translation of Theophrastus Paracelsus, 1633

☞ The alchemical processes seen here may be regarded as close to sorcery, given the raw material used; yet the methods are those of a chemistry laboratory. Epilepsy was inexplicable and fearful to the pre-modern mind – and its symptoms are still kept at a distance by using the terms 'grand mal' and 'petit mal' rather than describing them in the vernacular.

Soot coffee

Has cured many cases of ague, after 'everything else' failed; it is made as follows.

Soot scraped from a chimney (that from stove pipes does not do), 1 tablespoonful, steeped in water 1 pint, and settled with 1 egg beaten up in a little water, as for other coffee, with sugar and cream, 3 times daily with the meals, in place of other coffee.

It has come in very much to aid restoration in typhoid fever, bad cases of jaundice, dyspepsia, etc.

The Book You Want: How to cure everything, how to do everything, receipts for everything, John King 1885

☞ Though there is a long history of using soot as a medicinal ingredient, it may be carcinogenic.

Cinquefoil or five-leaved grass

The roots boiled in milk and drunk is a most effectual remedy, for all fluxes in man or woman, whether the whites, or reds, as also the bloody flux.

The English Physitian, Nicholas Culpeper, 1652

☞ 'White flux' was leucorrhoea, also known as 'the whites', a white discharge from the vagina; 'the reds', or 'red flux' was often used to mean the same as the 'bloody flux', but could be any discharge of blood from the anus. Cinquefoil is a recognized herbal treatment for both dysentery and leucorrhoea.

The black-thorn or sloe-bush

All the parts of the sloe-bush are binding, cooling and drying, and all effectual to stay bleeding at the nose and mouth, or any other place; the lask of the belly, or stomach, or the bloody flux, the too much abounding of women's courses, and helpeth to ease the pains in the sides, bowels, and guts, that come by over-much scowring; drink the decoction of the bark or the roots, or more usually the decoction of the berries either fresh or dried.

The English Physitian, Nicholas Culpeper, 1652

☞ The blackthorn, with its religious connection, was used against major maladies: 'lask', 'bloody flux' and visceral strains caused by too much heavy exercise ('scowring').

Ostrich fat

The fat of an ostrich is good for nervous parts, mollifies the hardness of the milt, assuages the nephritic pains (anointed).

The History of Animals as They are Useful in Physick and Chirurgery, John Schroder, 1659

☞ Nephritic pains were centred on the kidneys. Ostriches were not unknown in England at this time, and were believed to eat iron, which may lie behind a connection to the kidneys.

Liquid laudanum

From 14 to 15 drops, in any convenient vehicle, to be increased and diminished in proportion to the degree of pain and intervals of repetition. When judiciously administered, this is, no doubt, the most valuable medicine in the whole materia medica, and in certain stages, and with certain combinations, is advantageously employed in every disease incident to the human frame. It mitigates pain, induces sleep, allays inordinate action, and diminishes morbid irritability; hence it becomes an invaluable remedy obviating, and moderating symptomatic fevers from accidents. In spasmodic colic, it prevents inflammation of the bowels; and in all spasmodic affections it is more or less employed. In incurable diseases, where the sufferings of the patient are most excruciating, as in cancer, etc., it wonderfully alleviates the miseries, and renders the life of the patient tolerable.

If moderate doses of ten or twelve drops of liquid laudanum (which should always be begun with, says Dr Cullen) do not answer, they

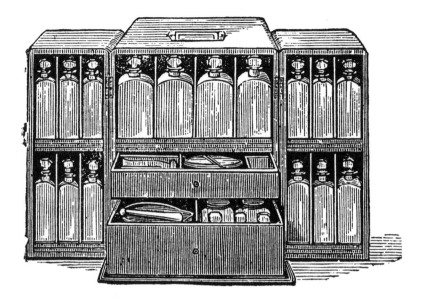

must be repeated and increased till the desired effect is obtained, and in this manner the doses of this drug may be pushed with safety to a very great length.

The Domestic Medical Guide, Richard Reece, 1803

☞ This is a typical indication of the taste for laudanum (basically opium), which saw much of the population of Britain stumbling through the first half of the nineteenth century in states ranging from hallucinatory creativity to drugged passivity. The willingness to increase dosage, and particularly the awareness that it could alleviate pain in hopeless conditions, must have allowed severely ill people to die relieved of pain.

Worms and snails

Both these are supposed to cool and cleanse the viscera. The latter, from their abounding with a viscid glutinous juice, are recommended as a restorative in consumptions; for this purpose they are directed to be boiled in milk [a longstanding recipe]; and thus managed they may possibly be of some service.

The New Dispensatory, William Lewis, 1778

☞ Current research in the West and medical applications in the East suggest that earthworms may have interesting antibacterial properties, and may help in the treatment of thrombosis. Snail mucus may have an application in antispasmodic treatment of the bronchial tree.

Upapa

[The lapwing] Is a melancholic bird, most nasty, living on worms found in dunghills. In physical use are 1. the flesh, 2. the feathers
 The virtues:
  1. The flesh and its decoction helps the colic by a propriety of its own.
  2. The feathers are said to assuage the head-ache (applied).

The History of Animals as They are Useful in Physick and Chirurgery, John Schroder, 1659

☞ 'Nasty' is a bit hard on the lapwing. And how would the feathers be applied to assuage a headache? Possibly by gentle stroking.

To distil oil of a man's excrement

Take the dung of a young sanguine child or man, as much as you will, and distil it twice in a limbeck of glass. This helpeth the canker, and mollifieth fistulas; comforteth those that are troubled with allopecia.

The Secrets of Physick and Philosophy, John Hester's translation of Theophrastus Paracelsus, 1633

☞ The only concession to modern sensibilities I can find in this is that, given the conditions mentioned, it was probably applied externally.

The web of spiders

The web astringes, conglutinates, and therefore is vulnerary, restraining blood and preventing inflammation. It is used not only outwardly, but also inwardly (boldly enough) to drive away feverish fits.

The History of Animals as They are Useful in Physick and Chirurgery, John Schroder, 1659

🢒 Spiders' webs have long been used for minor cuts.

Onions

For a nosebleed, put in an Onion.

The Garden of Health, William Langham, 1578

🢒 Onions were clearly of general use: 'Lethargy, put the juice of an onion into the nostrils. Urine stopped in agues, roast an onion, and apply it to the bladder.' Unfortunately Langham does not specify how it should be applied.

The oil of tilestones

It cureth the excoriation of the bladder, so well within as without (which is known by the biting or fretting of the yard) by anointing on the proper place. This helpeth the staying back of the urine, and hardness in the making of water.

The oil helpeth the passions of the ears proceeding of a cold cause, [such] as the deafness, the noise or hissing, and the flux of evil humors to the ears, by applying a fine linen cloth wet in it within the ears.

It bringeth forth the dead youngling by opening the mouths of the veins.

The Newe Jewell of Health, George Baker's translation of Conrad Gessner, 1576

🢒 The material here is a mixture of powdered brick and linseed oil; it is difficult to find any way that this could have relieved the stated conditions, especially a urinary tract infection. 'It bringeth forth the dead youngling' refers to the delivery of the dead foetus, thus avoiding the death of the mother too.

The garden parsnip

It nourisheth much, and is good and wholesome nourishment, but a little windy, whereby it is thought to procure bodily lust; but it fatteneth the body much if much used. It is conducible to the stomach and reins, and provoketh urine. But the wild parsnip hath a cutting, attenuating, cleansing and opening quality therein; it resisteth and helpeth the bitings of serpents, easeth pains and stitches in the sides, and dissolveth wind both in the stomach and bowels, which is the colic, and provoketh urine. The root is often used, but the seed much more.

The wild being better than the tame shows Dame Nature is the best physician.

The English Physitian, Nicholas Culpeper, 1652

🖙 The last sentence looks like another dig by Culpeper at the Royal College of Physicians. Richard Taverner, a sixteenth-century translator of the Bible, gives references to Plutarch, Cicero and Pythagoras connecting wind with lust, for which reason beans were frowned upon, as 'provoking impure humours'.

Sponge

The sponge is a kind of mushroom which grows to the rocks in the sea, of which there are two kinds. But though it is taken from the sea, authors have not yet determined in what class to place it: some thinking it to be neither vegetable, mineral nor animal; others that it participates of them all. Some again place it between animals and vegetables, and think it partakes of both of them, for that it has an active quality to dilate itself, and shrink up altogether, when in the sea, and therefore they will have it to be a plant animal; because in its nature it comes near both to that of an animal, and also to that of a plant.

The sponge is of an alkiline nature, and it is good against pains of the stomach, gripings in the bowels, and the colic; and is supposed to be a specific against the stone and gravel in the kidneys or bladder, or any obstruction in the urinary passages. The chief use of it is either in a powder calcined or crude.

A Compleat History of Drugs, Pierre Pomet, 1737

☞ Sponge is a useful item to have in any medicine cabinet, not just for cleaning. Pharmaceutical research starting from sponges led to the award of the 2010 Nobel Prize for Chemistry.

The hippopotamus or sea-horse

This is a four-footed animal, as big as an ox. The head is very thick, resembling more that of a calf than a horse; the mouth is a foot long, and the jaws are set with strong hard teeth, that will strike fire like a flint with steel, and are very proper to make artificial teeth with. The skin is so thick, that it is able to defend all manner of external violence, no bullet or spear being able to pierce it; the ashes thereof take away spots from the skin. The fat applied to the pulse or stomach, relieves fits of the ague and is emollient and nervous.

A Complete History of Drugs, Pierre Pomet, 1737

☞ No doubt many animals supplied the fat and skin that were passed off as coming from a hippopotamus. Hippopotamus fat here is considered relaxing and good for the nerves.

Corpus sine anima, a body without a soul

Roots of Florentine Orrice, musk, sugar, mixed to make a powder. It is of use to dissolve tartar in the lungs, help coughs and asthmas, etc, and takes away the stinking of the mouth or breath.

Bates' Dispensatory, translated and edited by William Salmon, 1694

☞ Salmon is clearly mystified by this recipe, as he states 'The name of this recipe is not stranger to me than the reason for which it was given. But that it will do something is certain.'

Mummy

Mummia is not much different from *Bitumen Indiacum*: for in Syria they embalm the corses of dead persons with *Bitumen Indiacum*; which embalming [material] with portions of the dead bodies is brought from thence, and it is called mummia; it is used against bruises, as well of the inward parts, as of the outwarde.

Approved Medicines and Cordiall Receiptes, Thomas Newton, 1580

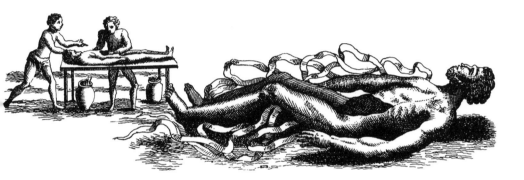

☞ That is to say that the pitch used to seal mummies was a medicinal material, but it was recognized that it would contain a certain seepage from the embalmed corpse with the bindings. Hall's translation of Lanfranc's *Chirurgerie* (1565) stated that 'Mumia' was a mixture of the 'embalming or spicery' of corpses along with aloes, myrrh and balsam and 'the fat and moisture of the corpse'.

In 1676, according to Gideon Harvey's *The Family-Physician and House-Apothecary*, a pound of this could be purchased for 5s 4d, compared to 1s for a pound of parsley seeds. By the eighteenth century the use of mummy had declined, as well as an awareness of exactly what it was, the 1716 *Pharmacopoeia Officinalis* stating that it was 'the flesh of carcasses which have been embalmed'. It had been superseded by 'parmasitty and other balsamics of the like kind'. 'Parmasitty' was an anglicization of *spermaceti*, used as an ointment base, indicating that 'mummia' could be used as a paste for holding more active ingredients.

Moss of an human skull

There is not any particular kind of moss that grows upon the human skull, nor does any moss by growing upon it acquire any particular virtues, whatever fanciful people may have imagined. In England, we commonly use the common ground moss, when it happens to run over an human skull, that has been laid by accident, or has been laid on purpose in its way; in other places, they use the sort of white moss, that grows upon our old apple-trees. Both these are in their own nature astringents, but they are as good if taken from trees, or off the ground, as if found upon these bones. They have been supposed good against disorders of the head, when gathered from the skull, but this is all fancy.

The Useful Family Herbal, John Hill, 1754

☞ Presumably the 'fancy' was the idea that the calmness of the moss creeping over a dead skull would have a similar effect on a live one. 'Skull-moss' was widely used in the seventeenth century, with moss being exported from Ireland to England and on to Germany.

A water of youth

This is so named the water of youth, in that it preserveth youth, and delivereth the person using it from sickness. Take of xyloaloes, of cloves, of ginger, of galingale, of cardomum, of cubebs, of grains of paradise, of rhubarb, of cinnamon, of nutmeg, of aloes, of calamus aromaticus, of mace, of each two drams, all these brought into a gross powder; searse [sift] diligently, adding to it the juice of celandine two pints, of sage, of bryony, of bugloss, and of fennell, of each half a pound, all these reduced into one, and distilled with the best white wine; of this distilled licquor drink every day in the summer time one spoonful, but in the winter two.

The Newe Jewell of Health, George Baker's translation
of Conrad Gessner, 1576

☞ 'Grains of paradise' were capsules of *Amomum melegueta*, imported from West Africa. What starts out as rather promising quickly becomes an extensive shopping list, but it was maybe worth a try.

Mithridates medicine against corrupt airs

Twenty leaves of rue, two fat figs, two walnuts, and a little salt; whosoever eateth of this composition shall be safe from all kind of venom that day.

The Widdowes Treasure, 1639

☞ A 'Mithridates medicine' was a powerful antidote, derived from the story that Mithridates, King of Pontus, took so many antidotes to preserve himself that he became proof against all known poisons. A 'Mithridate' thus became the name for any panacea.

The ultimate panacea

Salvator Winter, an Italian of the City of Naples, aged 98 years, yet, by the blessing of God, finds himself in health, and as strong as any one of fifty, as to the sensitive part – attributable to his *Elixir Vitae* which he always carries in his pocket in the day, and at night under his pillow. Good for everything including smallpox, measles, plague, dropsies, tympany and ruptures. This elixir hath such force and vigour, that if it were possible it would revive the dead, were it not a secret reserved to God only.

Handbill, *c.* 1700

☞ This gets close to the ultimate claim for a medicine. Winter cleverly recognises people's faith in medicines to the extent that they have to carry them about like talismans, their presence next to the body being part of their effect. 'Tympany' was tympanites, a swelling in the abdomen caused by gas, or abdominal dropsy, but the term was sometimes used to describe any morbid swelling or tumour.

Oil of frogs

Oleum Ranarum, oil of frogs. Ingredients: live frogs, 12, oil, olive.

Boil them for an hour, and express the oil.

It cures redness of the face and impetigo, helps erysipelas and gangrene, and is a specific against cancers.

Bates' Dispensatory, translated and edited by William Salmon, 1694

☞ Salmon's comment on this was 'It is a good thing for the intention, but in my opinion oil of toads is much before it, to all the purposes mentioned.'

How to cure the plague

THE MOST FEARED and perplexing disease of pre-modern times, plague (mainly bubonic, but also septicemic and pneumonic) resisted all attempts to treat it. It appeared that the only safe thing to do was to run away, but this often served to spread the disease.

To preserve your body from the infection of the plague

You shall take a quart of old ale, and after it hath risen upon the fire and hath been scummed, you shall put thereinto of birthwort, of angelica, and of celandine, of each half a handful, and boil them well therein; then strain the drink through a clean cloth and dissolve therein a dram of the best mithridate, as much ivory finely powdered and sifted, and six spoonfuls of dragon-water, then put it in a close glass. And every morning fasting take five spoonfuls thereof, and after bite and chew in your mouth the dried root of angelica, or smell a nosegay made of the raffled end of a ship-rope, and they will surely preserve you from infection.

The English Housewives' Household Physic, Gervase Markham, 1638

☞ Fear of the plague was such that it was worth knowing how to protect oneself against it as soon as an outbreak threatened. The power of angelica against the plague, and its name, were supposedly based on a divine visitation received by a medieval monk in plague-time. A mithridate was a universal antidote or panacea. Dragon-water was a popular medicine of the time.

To break the plague sore

Lay a roasted onion, also seethe a white lily root in milk, till it be as thick as a poultice, and lay it to the same; if these fail, lance the sore, and so draw it, and heal it with salves for botches or boils.

A Choice Manual of Rare and Select Secrets in Physick and Chyrurgery, Elizabeth Grey, 1653

☞ 'Botches' here are swellings. Sadly, lancing a plague bubo can cause more problems than it solves: a lanced bubo removes infected blood from the patient, but can infect anyone in the vicinity.

An experienced medicine for the plague

Take a cock, a chicken or a pullet, and pull all the feathers clean of the tail, so the rump may be bare, and then hold the rump or bare place to the sore, and immediately you shall see the cock, chicken or pullet gape, and labour for life, and in the end it will die; then take another cock, chicken or pullet again and do the like, and if the same die likewise, then take another, and do as aforesaid, and let the party grieved be applied therewith as aforesaid, as long as any of them do die.

A Rich Storehouse, or Treasurie for the Diseased, 1607

☞ The plague was intimately connected with animals; it was spread by rats, and given effective protection by a public health programme that advised people to kill cats and dogs. This remedy tries to force it back again into the animal world. The idea of drawing infection from a diseased person into an animal by direct contact is very old; there remains a persistent feeling that this is how poultices work, if only in the way we describe the action as 'drawing the poison/infection out'.

Against all manner of pestilence and plague

Take an onion and cut it overthwart [down the middle], then make a little hole in the middle of each piece, the which you shall fill with treacle, and lay the pieces together again, and wrap them in wet brown paper, and roast them in the hot embers; and being roasted enough, press out the juice of it, and give the patient to drink thereof a spoonful, and suddenly he shall feel himself better.

A Pretious Treasury, Or a New Dispensatory,
Salvator Winter and Francisco Dickinson, 1649

☞ Onion and treacle would both be helpful, but the claim that this would cure the plague is rather optimistic. However, onions do have anti-inflammatory and bacteriostatic properties, and treacle was originally used as an antidote to poison. Exactly the same remedy was given by William Langham in 1578.

An assured remedy for the plague, approved of throughout Venice in 1504

Take of a healthy male young child's water, fine treacle and aniseed water, of each a like quantity, mingle them, and give about a quarter of a pint or a little more at a time of it to the patient in the morning fasting, for three mornings altogether; this hath cured many.

A Brief Collection of Many Rare Secrets, Edward Fountaine, 1650

☞ Desperate times call for desperate measures; the fear-inducing power of the plague is seen in the credence given to a 150-year-old recipe involving drinking a child's urine.

Part of Nathaniel Hodges' treatment for the plague

When the physician is come, he ought to address the patient with cheerfulness, and blame those fears and melancholy apprehensions which give many over into the power of the distemper, by cutting off all hopes of recovery.

An emetic may be given in the infancy of the disease, where the stomach is loaded either by over-eating, or by a crowd of bad humours, or when there is a loathing, or a bitterness in the mouth; and amongst these remedies those are preferable which plentifully excite vomiting, without working also downwards.

Loimologia, Nathaniel Hodges, 1672

🙡 Hodges wrote his account of the 1665 Great Plague in London having stayed in the city and ministered to the sick throughout the epidemic. His is the best witness we have to the disease at that time. This passage is from an extensive remedy for the plague, with several stages of treatment. He did however believe that the best treatment was 'the oriental bezoar'.

Hodges had a remedy 'for the Richer Sort' which contained pearl, white amber, bezoar stone and unicorn's horn, but he was aware that what was needed in the case of London in 1665 was a treatment for the common people rather than the wealthy, who could after all afford to leave the pestilential city.

Of the pestilential fever of the years 1665, 1666

After the sick person hath been let blood in his bed, let him be covered all over with cloths, and his forehead bound about with a piece of woollen cloth, and then if he doth not vomit, let some medicine to procure sweat be exhibited to him, [such] as:

Take Treacle of Andromachus half a dram, Electuary de Ovo, one scruple, powder of crabs-claws compound twelve grains, cochineal eight grains, saffron four grains, with a sufficient quantity of the juice of kernes [corn] to make a bolus, which must be repeated every sixth hour, drinking after it six spoonfuls of the following Julep.

Take Carduus Benedictus water, and compound scordium water, of each four ounces; distilled treacle water, two ounces; syrup of clove-gilliflowers, one ounce; mix them for a Julep.

After the breaking forth of a swelling, I durst not open a vein; let the sick person keep his bed four and twenty hours after the sweating is over, and diligently avoid all manner of cold, suffering his shirt to dry of itself upon his body. Let him drink nothing but what is hot, and still persist in the use of sage posset; next morning let him take the common purging potion.

The Compleat Method of Curing Almost All Diseases,
Thomas Sydenham, 1694

☞ The whole business of being infected and of nursing the sick during the plague must have been appalling; we can only imagine the mixture of smells. The treacle and the electuary were both general medicinal mixtures. 'Carduus Benedictus water' was made from a thistle, while 'scordium' was the water-germander, used to induce sweating.

A treatment for the plague

You shall give then three or four mornings altogether one dram and a half of our *Pillule Aquilone*, and once a day you shall anoint all his body with our Balsano Artificiato [artificial balsam], because it killeth that poison and preserveth the body. Also you shall open the sores quickly that the matter may come forth, and when they are broken you shall put therein our caustic once only, because it purgeth it divinely.

A Joyfull Jewel, T. Hill's translation of Leonardo Fioravanti (1579)

☞ The original text spells 'caustic' as 'cowstick', which is a little disturbing. The idea here is to clean the pores so that all the poison can come out. Noticeable here also is the marketing of proprietary medicines to the reader.

Plague, hot

Drink as much powder of the root [of dog-fennel] as will lie on a crown-coin with vinegar, but in the cold plague with wine. Drink the juice of a handful of it with a pint of Malmesey against the ague, the plague, and to comfort nature every morning.

The Garden of Health,
William Langham, 1578

To 'comfort nature every morning' with a pint of wine might not be a bad way to face any day.

AFTERWORD

BUT IN ORDER to avoid diseases, a strict regard should be paid to temperance and regularity, first in cleanliness of apparel, diet and habitation; taking exercise as much as possible in the open air; to make choice of that food which is wholesome and not over kept, as in animal food and fish which hath been kept above three days is turning to putrescency, and creates diseases, therefore should be avoided in that state; also bad water, which is corrupt through stagnation, should not be used, as it generates scurvies, and cutaneous eruptions; all night air, late hours, wet feet, damp floors and linen; also any of the depressing passions have a great influence over the body, such as grief, despair, anger, fear, envy, etc. But to conclude, those who live philosophically, live temperately, religiously and wisely, seldom want a physician; but when that is the case, by taking the disease in time, it is easily deprived of its force and soon becomes eradicated; as on the contrary when the disease is become, through neglect, rooted in the habit, it not only weakens the constitution but encreases the expense, which must naturally arise from a further supply of medicines.

The Family Physician,
Edward Bullman, 1789

A BRIEF GLOSSARY

AGUE Fever

ALEMBIC/LIMBECK A flask with a neck bending downwards to one side

BEZOAR A hard mass, usually of hair, forming in the stomach; oriental
    goats' bezoars were prized for their supposed healing properties

BLISTER A plaster producing blistering

BLOODY FLUX Dysentery

BOLUS A ball, larger than a pill

BRAY, BRUISE, STAMP To crush

CATAPLASM Plaster

CHYRURGEON Surgeon

CHYRURGERY Surgery

CLYSTER Enema

COPPERAS A proto-sulphate, usually of iron

DECOCT To concentrate by boiling

DISTIL To extract a liquid, either by boiling and condensation, or through
    gravity

DROPSY An accumulation of fluid in the body

ELECTUARY Sweet conserve or paste

EMETIC Stimulating vomiting

FALLING SICKNESS Epilepsy

FLUX/LASK Diarrhoea

HARTSHORN The shavings of horn, used to produce oil of hartshorn,
    spirit of hartshorn (aqueous solution of ammonia) and salt of
    hartshorn (sal ammoniac, or ammonium chloride)

IMPOSTUME Inflammation, boil

LIGHTS Lungs

LYE An alkaline solution prepared from ashes

MATRIX/MOTHER Uterus or womb

MATRASS A flask

MILT Spleen

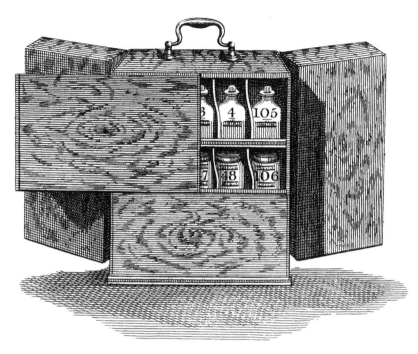

PALSY Paralysis and/or tremor

PHYSICK Medicine

QUINSY/SQUINANCY Throat infection

RECTIFY To purify by repeated distillation

REINS The kidneys, but 'running of the reins' was gonorrhoea

SEETHE To boil

SMART Pain

SPIRITS OF SALT Hydrochloric acid

SPIRITS OF WINE *Aqua vitae*, or aqueus solution of ethanol

STYPTIC Constricting the tissues or blood vessels

TERMS, FLOWERS, MENSES AND COURSES Menstrual flow

TROCHISCES Lozenges

VITRIOL A metal sulphate; blue (or Roman), green, red and white vitriol
were sulphates respectively of copper, iron, cobalt and zinc

WEN A hard lump under the skin, a sebaceous cystic tumour

YARD/CODS Male genitals

LIST OF ILLUSTRATIONS